Contributing Authors

Stephen R. Carden, EMT-P
Program Director, EMS
Joint Hospital Planning Council of
    Greater Bridgeport
Bridgeport, Connecticut;
ACLS Instructor

Mark Forgues, EMT-P, MEd
Director of Education
Boston Medical Education Group
Ashby, Massachusetts;
ACLS Affiliate Faculty

Robert Howell, RN, PA-C
Veterans Administration Medical Center
    (VAMC)
West Haven, Connecticut;
ACLS Affiliate Faculty

Steven Mercer, REMT-P
Iowa Department of Public Health EMS
    Division
State Training Coordinator
Des Moines, Iowa;
ACLS Instructor

Jean K. Pals, RN-C
Consult/Liaison Nurse
Geriatrics and Extended Care Service
Brockton/West Roxbury VAMC
Brockton, Massachusetts;
ACLS Instructor

Joseph Sciammarella, MD, FACP, EMT-P
Director, Division of EMS
Medical Director Suffolk County EMS
Suffolk County Department of Health
    Services
Yaphank, New York;
ACLS Affiliate Faculty

Dorothy Turnbull, MD, FACEP
Chief, Department of Emergency Medicine
Stamford Hospital
Stamford, Connecticut;
Vice Chairperson
ACLS/PALS Committee
Connecticut Heart Association;
ACLS Affiliate Faculty

Elizabeth M. Wertz, RN, EMT-P
Manager, Life Support Training Center
Allegheny General Hospital
Pittsburgh, Pennsylvania;
ACLS Affiliate Faculty

Easy ACLS

Advanced Cardiac Life Support Preparatory Manual

Editor

Andrew L. Wi_____ ___D, FACP
ACLS Affiliate Faculty
_____ _____ ___assachusetts Affiliate;
ACLS Medical Director, Bro___on/West Roxbury VAMC
_____ Massachusetts
_____ Medicine
Harvard Medi___ School
Boston, Mass_____tts

James L. Perusas, ____P
ACLS Nation_____
_____ttee
Americ_____onnecticut Affiliate;
_____pital
_____ Center

thors

Don Greswell Ltd. London, N.21 Cat. No. 1207   DG 02242/71

_____ers
____lon

Editorial, Sales, and Customer Service Offices

Jones and Bartlett Publishers
One Exeter Plaza
Boston, MA 02116
1-800-832-0034
1-617-859-3900

Jones and Bartlett Publishers International
7 Melrose Terrace
London W6 7RL
England

Library of Congress Cataloging-in-Publication Data

Easy ACLS: advanced cardiac life support preparatory manual/
    editors, Andrew D. Weinberg, James L. Paturas: with eight
    contributing authors.
         p.   cm.
      Includes index.
      ISBN 0-86720-819-8
        1. Cardiovascular emergencies—Treatment. 2. CPR (First aid)
    3. Cardiac arrest—Treatment. 4. Arrhythmia—Treatment.
    I. Weinberg, Andrew David. II. Paturas, James L.
      [DNLM: 1. Heart Diseases—therapy. 2. Resuscitation—methods.
    3. Life Support Care—methods. WG 205 E13 1995]
    RC675.E27 1995
    616.1'2025—dc20
DNLM/DLC
for Library of Congress   95-3411
                                           CIP

Vice President and Publisher: Clayton E. Jones
Production Editor: Anne S. Noonan
Manufacturing Buyer: Dana L. Cerrito
Typesetting: LeGwin Associates
Editorial Service: Colophon
Cover Design: Marshall Hendrichs
Printing and Binding: Courier

Printed in the United States of America
99 98 97 96 95   10 9 8 7 6 5 4 3 2 1

Contents

Quick Reference Charts

1. BCLS Performance Guidelines

2. ACLS Algorithms

3. ACLS Adult Drug Chart

1 Introduction and Overview

The teaching of Advanced Cardiac Life Support (ACLS) has now extended into every facet of emergency medicine and many medical school curriculums. The latest revision of ACLS standards, which resulted from the final reports of the 1992 National Conference on Cardiopulmonary Resuscitation and Emergency Cardiac Care, represents the latest scientific information available on the optimal approach to the management of emergency cardiopulmonary events. All revised standards for cardiopulmonary resuscitation (CPR) and ACLS were published in the *Journal of the American Medical Association* (JAMA), October 28, 1992 (vol. 268, no. 16).

The organization of information and logical interventions for such emergencies are an integral part of the ACLS curriculum. The use of "mega code/case-based teaching stations" to simulate both cardiopulmonary arrests and other critical cardiovascular conditions help participants obtain vital practice employing ACLS standards. Teamwork, one of the most difficult aspects in running an effective code, remains an important teaching objective.

This book is intended to serve as a study guide not only for the new algorithms and medication recommendations but also for taking the American Heart Association's (AHA) ACLS Provider course in general. It is *not* intended to serve as a substitute for taking CPR, ACLS, or pediatric ACLS (PALS) courses, nor will it replace the new AHA textbook, which greatly expands the scientific basis for the material presented here. It is important to stress that each patient must continue to have his or her care individualized by the medical team; adjustments in medications and all interventions must be tailored depending on the clinical circumstances that exist at the time of the emergency and the ongoing response to treatment.

The probability of survival after a cardiopulmonary event declines rapidly with each minute of arrest or compromise of circulation. Basic CPR can slow this decline, but unless the underlying pathology is recognized (e.g., ventricular tachycardia, ventricular fibrillation, asystole) and correctly treated, successful recovery will rarely be possible. The majority of successful resuscitations depend on early defibrillation, as an initial rhythm disturbance of ventricular fibrillation causes 80% to 90% of all nontraumatic cardiac arrests.

ACLS should be thought of as a *continuum* of evaluation, treatment, and ongoing monitoring. The ACLS recommendations offer the healthcare provider general clinical guidelines for a variety of cardiopulmonary emergencies, including the management of severe hypothermia. The algorithms and drug dosages recommended are to be utilized in the appropriate clinical setting, but the code team must be able to change and modify treatment strategies for each patient as the clinical picture and response to intervention evolves during the code.

The code team, under the direction of the *team leader,* must function smoothly as codes can take unexpected and unpredictable courses at times. A capable team leader must be a good organizer and supervisor of the team members' individual and collective performance. The primary characteristic of a good team leader is that he or she must exhibit the leadership necessary to maximize appropriate treatment and minimize confusion during the code. The team leader should always communicate his or her observations and diagnoses to the team throughout the code and maintain an attitude that is conducive for members to make suggestions regarding further treatment strategies. It is important to avoid letting egos get in the way of a successful code. This, perhaps, remains one of the more difficult points to teach in an ACLS provider course.

Specialized procedures, such as intubation and central line placement, must be performed by qualified personnel. When such personnel are not yet at the site of the emergency, ventilation with a bag-mask unit and peripheral intravenous (IV) approaches should be employed.

Learning ACLS and feeling comfortable with the new material adopted by the AHA in 1992 takes time and practice. However, with the new recommendations and treatment strategies now being taught in the ACLS Provider Course, code teams now have more comprehensive methods with which to approach cardiopulmonary arrests and other medical emergencies. We believe the reader will find this book helpful not only for taking an ACLS course but also for learning how to run more successful resuscitations.

The editors wish to thank the AHA for allowing us to reproduce its algorithms in this book.

Notes

2 Goals and Objectives

The primary objective of this manual is to offer a reference guide and resource to those participating in either an initial or a refresher ACLS provider course. This text has been prepared for use by health-care providers who are required to maintain proficiency in adult ACLS.

The information contained in this manual conforms to the standards established by the American Heart Association Emergency Cardiac Care Committee. The ACLS guidelines are reprinted by permission of the Emergency Cardiac Care Committee of the American Heart Association as originally published in the October 28, 1992, edition of the *Journal of the American Medical Association.* This text is meant to serve as a quick reference to the material presented in the *AHA ACLS Provider Textbook.* For those participants who do not have the time to read the entire AHA text, this book will serve to highlight and emphasize those points most critical to understanding the ACLS material and passing the course. This book will also help individuals review those areas of the ACLS curriculum they might feel weak in and thus pinpoint where further work is required before attending the ACLS course.

The treatment algorithms were developed by the AHA primarily for use in the hospital setting. Emergency medical technicians (EMTs) and paramedics should understand some of the restrictions of their use for prehospital care and adjust them accordingly after discussion with local physician medical control.

It is not our intention to present this manual as a replacement for the ACLS textbook published by the AHA but rather to offer an additional resource. In preparing this book, the editors and authors have attempted to make it as user friendly as possible. Although the chapters may go by different titles, they are consistent with the core material required by the AHA for use in the ACLS program. This includes information for both the instructional and evaluation (testing) components of the ACLS provider course.

It is important to note that there will be a new emphasis on *case-based teaching*, rather than using the traditional subject-based format. Patient case scenarios will be used to illustrate the entire spectrum of management of the patient described, including pharmacological intervention, airway management, required electrical intervention, and postresuscitation stabilization techniques. Special emphasis will be placed on managing the first 10 minutes of ventricular fibrillation (VF). There will be a total of nine core ACLS cases, which will have an algorithm accompanying each case. These nine case scenarios are

- Respiratory arrest
- Pulseless VF/ventricular tachycardia (VT) treated with an automated external defibrillator
- VF/VT refractory to initial defibrillation
- Pulseless electrical activity (includes the "old" electromechanical dissociation group)
- Asystole
- Acute myocardial infarction (MI)
- Bradycardia
- Stable tachycardia
- Unstable tachycardia

Supplemental materials may also be offered for ACLS courses with *experienced providers*. These areas include the additional following case scenarios:

- Hypotension/shock/acute pulmonary edema
- Drowning
- Hypothermia
- Cardiac arrest due to trauma
- Electrical shock/electrocution/lightning strike
- Stroke
- Ethical aspects of resuscitation
- Psychological aspects of resuscitation
- Phased-response resuscitation

Because this text is developed as a self-study tool, you will find examples of test questions and *patient case-based teaching scenarios* included. These will be useful for the ACLS provider student as well as for the ACLS instructor.

General Considerations

The ACLS guidelines and the educational process for teaching them are always evolving, both for the student and for the instructor. There will now be more emphasis placed on reasonable remediation rather than simple passing and failing of the ACLS course.

Besides the obvious clinical information that an ACLS course participant must master, there are a number of other nonclinical characteristics that are required for successful completion of the course. If you were to dissect the anatomy of a "good ACLS code situation," some of the critical components of its success would be based on the clinical expertise of the individuals, clearly defined leadership, the ability of each individual to work as part of a team, and the art of effective communication. Leadership can be defined in many ways, but, in essence, it is the ability to influence others to carry out assigned tasks and directives and to perform as required according to job specifications. There is nothing as important as the need to delegate authority in an emergency situation. In order for directives to be carried out, each member of the team must understand his or her job and believe that that person can carry out the assigned tasks.

An individual learns to lead by following the examples set by others (and, of course, being competent in the area being taught) and remaining sensitive to the cues sent forth by other leaders. Before the ACLS team leader can begin to exercise authority over others at the code, he or she must consider his or her own reactions to authority. A person who does not come to grips with his or her own emotional reactions to being "the leader," will find it difficult to employ his or her authority prudently and productively with others.

Another important component of managing the code involves effective communication. Communication is a form of influence. It involves a relationship in which all individuals play distinct but complementary roles. The major purpose of effective communication is the transmission of information.

The Apprehension Factor

Webster's Ninth New Collegiate Dictionary describes the word *apprehension* as "suspicion or fear, especially of future evil." Others would describe it as taking an ACLS provider course with a special focus on mega code/case-based teaching station testing.

As you prepare to attend the ACLS provider course, you can reduce your tension level through early preparation. This will involve practicing your critical intervention skills (e.g., airway management, defibrillation) as well as reviewing electrocardiogram (ECG) interpretation, emergency cardiac pharmacology, and ACLS algorithms.

In addition, knowledge of the dynamics of the teaching/testing environment will also contribute to a successful outcome. This means that the attitude and demeanor you exhibit during your attendance at an ACLS course will leave an impression on the faculty. Any negative bias that you are aware of from previous ACLS courses should be dealt with prior to attending the course again. If you are not able to deal with these issues, your feelings may be "telegraphed" to the faculty.

Remember, the ultimate goal of an educational experience is to share information and help the participants achieve successful completion of the program. In general, most ACLS instructors have not forgotten what it is like to be in your position and, as such, will do everything they can to make your experience meaningful and nonthreatening. Even when they review your strengths and weaknesses, it is done in an effort to correct deficiencies and to build up your confidence. In all likelihood, you are not the only one who is having high anxiety.

When you enter the course, show confidence where appropriate, ask questions about any of the material you do not understand, and talk through the practice skill stations. Don't forget to exhibit leadership characteristics during the mega code/case-based teaching stations and *never panic*!

Summary

This textbook is designed to enhance your preparation for participating in the ACLS course. It is our recommendation that you read the ACLS textbook published by the AHA, take some time to practice with the written pretests, and practice your intervention skills. We hope that this preparatory text will be a valuable resource to you and will help to give you a greater understanding of the primary components of the ACLS program.

Notes

3 So You Are About to Take (or Retake) an ACLS Course

Objectives

1. Distinguish the advantages of all emergency health-care providers becoming certified in ACLS.
2. Discuss the best methods to prepare for taking an ACLS course.

Confronting the Inevitable

So you want to take an ACLS course or maybe it is simply your turn to undergo this rigorous training exercise? Why is it important for you to learn ACLS? First, you will be exposed to a training program that incorporates national standards for cardiac care. This simply means that representatives from various groups have met on many occasions, looked at the research, collaborated, and determined the best way to care for a patient with a cardiac emergency. You immediately benefit from this multidisciplinary wealth of knowledge and experience. Available to them were all the tricks of the trade so that they could establish standards by which others would be judged or held accountable.

Second, you benefit from the experience, or inexperience if that is the case, of the other students in the class. Learning takes place even during the breaks, especially if the students are from a mixture of backgrounds, such as paramedics, critical care, cardiology, anesthesiology, or emergency medicine. Many of them may also be quite anxious, and a camaraderie develops among complete strangers brought together for the sole purpose of passing this class. Additionally, some of the course material presented may be updated from the last time you took the course and these changes are important to understand.

How to Prepare

What can you do to prepare? Most importantly, stop listening to other people's horror stories and develop your own game plan. Obtain the written materials as far in advance as possible. Take time to read the book.

Are you studying the old guidelines and algorithms or the new ones? What is the date on your materials? What is the date on the textbook? The AHA performs updates approximately every five years, so make sure your information has the most recent dating available.

Do you have a current basic cardiac life support (BCLS) provider card? Many people assume that BCLS is part of the ACLS course. It is true that there is a BCLS station, but this is for the instructor to verify your BCLS skills; it is not to issue you a new card. You should have a current BCLS provider card *prior* to taking an ACLS provider or renewal course.

Lectures

It is important that you read the book and any handouts provided to you before the first day of class. The lectures do not go into great detail on every chapter and some reading before the course will help you identify any weak areas you might have and thus questions you may wish to ask. Additionally, there are many study guides that can give a concise summary of the current ACLS material and may prove useful in reviewing a great deal of material in a short period of time. Use whatever method is easiest for you when reading. Some people like to make an outline of the information in each chapter. Others prefer to use a highlighter and emphasize key points. Just remember to bring your book and notes to class with you for reference.

Teaching Skill Stations

For the mega code/case-based teaching station and/or therapeutic modalities station, it will help significantly if you either know the algorithms or are at least familiar with them before you walk through the door. This will help you to follow along through the stations and you will not have to study quite as hard the night before the evaluation stations. In addition, notes are permitted at these stations during the teaching.

Finally, you should know how to read an ECG before taking this course. This program does *not* teach you the intricacies of interpreting ECGs. Many individuals may have come into the course expecting three weeks of critical care classes to be taught in just two days! It doesn't happen that way! If you are not proficient on ECG interpretation you should plan on spending several weeks before the course reviewing any difficult areas so the course can serve more as a review for you than as a teaching session.

Evaluation Stations

You must know the algorithms as well as be able to recognize ECG rhythms on the monitor. Take your time and feel free to ask questions if you don't understand what the evaluator is saying or asking you to do.

Remember, you are role playing. It is important to tell the evaluator what you are thinking. For example, in the mega code/case-based teaching station when you are initially assessing the patient, ask, "Is the airway open? Is he breathing? Do I feel a pulse?" As you are treating this "patient" again explain what you are doing, "I am checking his pulse again. Is it still present?"

Some training sites will have equipment available and ask you to use it as you routinely would do. Others ask you to verbally go through the exercise. If the equipment is available, use it to better simulate a live situation. Use the stethoscope to listen for breath sounds after the intubation. Actually put the blood pressure cuff on the manikin's arm and pump it up. Use the equipment to make the scenario as real as possible.

Written Exam

The test is comprised of 50 multiple-choice questions. Don't perform a microscopic exam on each question and "what if" it to death. Read the questions and potential answers. Choose the best possible answer from those given on the piece of paper. One trick-of-the-trade is to run through the written exam without hesitation and answer those questions that you know. After you have completed the exam, go back and tackle the questions that gave you some difficulty.

Don't over study in one area. Stick to the basics: Learn the drugs and why they are used. Know what situation requires which medications. Know the fundamental drug dosages. This all sounds difficult, but if you learn one group at a time the mountain can be climbed.

ECG Exam

Many courses require the passing of a written ECG recognition test. If so, there should be a pretest to familiarize yourself with what is expected on the final exam. The course director will provide the specific testing requirements of your particular course. You may wish to follow the same method for the ECG written test. That is, run through the exam without hesitation and answer those questions that you know immediately. After you have completed the exam, go back and tackle the questions that gave you some difficulty.

Summary

In summary, taking or retaking an ACLS course can be a major challenge for some and a breeze for others. Prepare for your level of skill and expertise. Don't let your ego get in the way of studying or asking a friend or colleague to help you prepare for the course. In this way, you can give the course your best effort, being more knowledgeable and better prepared to deal with the business of saving lives.

Notes

4 Update and Overview on Basic Cardiac Life Support

Objectives

1. Describe some of the changes the AHA has made to BCLS protocols.
2. Understand the theory of active compression-decompression CPR.

Introduction

In the 30 years since standards for the teaching of BCLS were developed, many advances in the emergency care of cardiac arrest victims have been made. Since electrical reversal of ventricular fibrillation by use of externally applied electrodes was described in 1956, this has challenged the medical community to develop a method of sustaining ventilation and circulation long enough to bring the defibrillator to the patient's aid. In 1960, closed-chest cardiac compression was described, ushering in the modern era of CPR.

BCLS is important for the ACLS student to understand as it is an early link in the chain of survival. By adequately oxygenating the patient in a timely manner through prompt initiation of ventilations and compressions, you are optimizing the patient's chance of survival and for a better neurologic outcome. Also, maintaining current BCLS certification is a requirement for all ACLS courses.

In 1966, the first conference on CPR was sponsored by the National Academy of Sciences–National Research Council with the main emphasis on the teaching and dissemination of CPR standards to medical and other allied health professionals. By 1973, the AHA had recommended that this training be extended to the general public. At the same time, the roles of various other agencies, such as the American Red Cross, were defined in relation to the training of citizens. In 1983 and 1985, the AHA recognized the need for pediatric and child resuscitations, and recommendations were proposed and endorsed by the American Academy of Pediatrics.

Cardiovascular disease accounts for nearly 1 million deaths in the United States annually, including approximately 500,000 deaths due to coronary disease, a majority of which are sudden deaths. Approximately two thirds of sudden deaths due to coronary disease take place outside the hospital and usually occur within two hours after onset of symptoms.

Even with the declining death rate from coronary heart disease (CHD) over the past several decades (30% decrease in CHD from 1979 to 1989), sudden death related to coronary artery disease (CAD) is still the most prominent medical emergency in the United States today. It may be possible that a large number of these deaths due to CAD are preventable by prompt action to provide rapid entry into the emergency medical service (EMS) system, quick beginning of CPR, and early defibrillation.

Because the majority of sudden deaths caused by cardiac arrest occur before hospitalization, it is important that the general public or community be recognized as a target audience for the training and dissemination of information. The AHA has and will continue to educate the public concerning their responsibility in the chain of survival, including detection and modification of risk factors, recognition of signs of impending cardiac events, and knowledge of BCLS techniques.

It is understood that CPR alone is of limited usefulness in the actual saving of a cardiac arrest victim's life, but it is considered an integral part of the chain of survival: early access, early CPR, early defibrillation, and early ACLS. What CPR does is "buy the rescuer a nominal amount of time" to support cardiopulmonary circulation until ACLS-trained persons and equipment can arrive on the scene. This is best realized if defibrillation or other definitive modes of care can be initiated within 8 to 10 minutes. If CPR or the other definitive modes of care are delayed, the chain of survival is broken, brain tissue is irreversibly damaged from hypoxia, and there is resulting severe neurologic deficit or death.

This brings us to the point, raised by many, of the efficacy and appropriateness of CPR in certain instances and among certain populations. Undoubtedly, BCLS training classes have improved the techniques of CPR practitioners in clinical settings, but, to date, there are no empirical data to suggest that these courses have improved patient outcomes. In fact, it has been reported that most participants in BCLS training programs, medical and lay people alike, do not retain the skills and knowledge obtained for more than six months despite intensive training sessions.

Survival to hospital discharge has been documented as low as 0% to 3% in studies reported in 1991 and 1992 among several different populations. Higher survival in hospital discharge rates have been reported, but the varied outcomes can be attributed to several factors, such as inconsistent inclusion criteria, multisystem disease in hospitalized populations, variations in EMS systems, adequacy of CPR provided, and interval from arrest to provision of ACLS. Nonetheless, the reports of low survival rates does question, perhaps, the overall value of CPR. The effectiveness of CPR should be evaluated just as the effectiveness of other medical interventions is evaluated. The AHA Guidelines[1] (as published in the October 28, 1992, JAMA supplement) do suggest appropriate applications of, and mechanisms for withholding CPR along with support for termination of resuscitative efforts in the field. These issues need to be discussed with patients and/or family members.

Like the previous recommendations, these represent a consensus of experts from a variety of disciplines. The recommendations of the 1992 Conference on Cardiopulmonary Resuscitation and Emergency Cardiac Care do not represent broad changes and are considered the most effective and the most easily teachable that current knowledge and experience can provide.

The chain of survival (early access, early CPR, early defibrillation, and early advanced care) had one weak link until recently—the early defibrillation. It has been noted that 80% to 90% of adults with sudden nontraumatic cardiac arrest are found to be in ventricular fibrillation when the initial ECG is obtained. We are all aware that the only real definitive treatment for this arrhythmia is defibrillation; thus, the need for early access into the EMS system to provide the patient with trained personnel and equipment to perform the defibrillation. There have been documented improved survival rates of patients with cardiac arrest in communities with no pre-hospital ACLS, but early defibrillation (7% to 26% in Washington state and 3% to 19% in Iowa).

With the above principle in mind, the Emergency Cardiac Care (ECC) Committee has integrated into the BCLS protocol for rescuers who come upon an adult who has collapsed and/or who is unresponsive to activate the EMS system immediately. They then are to return to the victim for assessment of the ABCs and begin CPR as indicated. It is felt by the ECC Committee that **Phone first for adults only** is a truly lifesaving act.

However, in the pediatric age group, the most common cause of arrest is primary respiratory arrest or an obstructed airway. Ventricular fibrillation in children is uncommon. Consequently, the recommendation for pediatric emergencies is to assess the patient and provide approximately one minute of rescue support before activating the EMS system.

Recovery Position

If a victim resumes breathing and regains a pulse during or following resuscitation, the rescuer should continue to help maintain a patent airway. The rescuer should then place the victim in the recovery position by rolling him or her onto the side so that the head, shoulders, and torso move simultaneously without twisting. This will prevent the tongue, the most common cause of airway obstruction in the unconscious person, from falling back into the oropharynx area and obstructing the airway. If trauma or injury is suspected, the victim should not be moved.

A summary of the BCLS changes is found in Table 4.1.

Ambu Cardiopump

Recently, a comparison of active compression-decompression CPR using a hand-held suction device (Ambu CardioPump) versus regular

■ **Table 4.1**   **Summary of Changes in Basic Cardiac Life Support (BCLS)
Techniques as Published in the October 28, 1992, Issue of JAMA**

Skill/Issue	Old Guidelines (1986)	New Guidelines (1992)
Activation of EMS system	*Adult, child and infant:* Activate EMS system after 1 minute of CPR or rescue breathing	*Adult:* Activate the EMS system immediately after determining unresponsiveness. EMS activation prior to any resuscitation attempts. *Child and infant:* Same as old guidelines. 1 minute of CPR or rescue breathing prior to EMS activation if the rescuer is alone.
Adult rescue breathing rate	Once every five seconds	Once every five to six seconds
Adult rescue breathing duration	1 to 1.5 seconds per breath; deep, full breaths	1.5 to 2 seconds per breath to make the chest rise. **Slow, full** breaths reduce air from entering the stomach (preventing gastric distension).
Position of unconscious, breathing victim (non-traumatic)	Not mentioned.	A recovery position is described: Victim rolled on side, keeping torso from twisting.
Airway	Gastric distension can be minimized by keeping the airway open during exhalation (e.g., during two-rescuer CPR)	
Depth of compressions for infant and child	*Child*: 1 to 1.5 inches *Infant*: 0.5 to 1.0 inch	Depths remain the same
Foreign-body airway obstruction procedure: Adult and Child [a]	*Conscious:* Abdominal thrusts until object expelled or victim becomes unconscious	*Conscious:* Up to five abdominal thrusts administered. Reassess victim's status and rescuer's technique. Repeat as necessary.

■ **Table 4.1**   (con't)

Skill/Issue	Old Guidelines (1986)	New Guidelines (1992)
Foreign-body airway obstruction procedure: Adult and Child [a] (con't)	*Unconscious:* Six to ten abdominal thrusts, finger sweep (adult), remove visible object (child), attempt two breaths. If unsuccessful in clearing airway, repeat sequence.	*Unconscious:* Administer up to five abdominal thrusts, finger sweep (adult), remove visible object (child), attempt two breaths. If unsuccessful in clearing airway, repeat sequence.
Foreign-body airway obstruction procedure: Infant [a]	*Conscious:* Cycle of four back blows, four chest thrusts until object is dislodged or infant becomes unconscious.	*Conscious:* Administer up to five (5) back blows and up to five chest thrusts, mouth check for object. If unsuccessful in clearing airway, repeat sequence until object is cleared or infant becomes unconscious.
	Unconscious: Cycle of four back blows, four chest thrusts, mouth check, remove visible object, two breaths. If unsuccessful in clearing airway, repeat sequence.	*Unconscious:* Administer up to five back blows and up to five chest thrusts, mouth check for object, remove visible object, two breaths. If unsuccessful in clearing airway, repeat sequence.

[a] Attempt to ventilate in foreign-body airway obstruction in all sequences for all ages: Every time the first breath does not go in, reposition the victim's head and try to give a second breath. Obviously if trauma is suspected or evident, the jaw thrust without head tilt would be used.

CPR of cardiac arrests occurring in the hospital was conducted.[2] The study concluded that the use of the CardioPump improved the rate of initial resuscitation, survival at 24 hours, and neurologic outcome after in-hospital cardiac arrest. However, it was pointed out that larger trials will be required to assess any benefits in terms of long-term survival. The AHA has not endorsed the use of this device for CPR at the present time.

It is important for the student taking the ACLS course to realize that by increasing the ability to deliver improved oxygenation to the brain during basic CPR, it is possible for the patient to then be in a better neurologic position for ACLS resuscitation.See Table 4.2.

■ **Table 4.2**   **BCLS Quick Reference Chart: Performance Guidelines**

Performance	Infant (≤ 1 Year)	Child (1 to 8 Years)	Adult
Airway	Head tilt/chin lift (If trauma suspected, jaw thrust)	Same	Same
Breathing	2 breaths at 1 to 1½ sec/breath	Same	2 breaths at 1½ to 2 sec/breath
Compress with	2 fingers	Heel of 1 hand	2 hands (heel) stacked
Position	1 finger's width below inter-mammary line	Locate end of sternum with middle finger, index finger next to it, heel of hand beside it	Same (except heel of other hand beside it and stack hands)
Depth of compression	½ to 1 inch	1 to 1½ inches	1½ to 2 inches
Pulse check	Brachial	Carotid	Carotid
Rate of compression	At least 100/min	100/min	80 to 100/min
Ratio of compressions to ventilations	5:1	5:1	15:2 (1-person CPR) 5:1 (2-person CPR)
Rescue breathing	1 breath every 3 sec (20 per min)	Same	1 breath every 5 to 6 sec (10 to 12 per min)
Foreign-body airway obstruction	Back blows and chest thrusts	Abdominal thrusts	Same

References

1. Guidelines for Cardiopulmonary Resuscitation and Emergency Cardiac Care. *JAMA* 1992;268:2171–2302.
2. Cohen TJ, Goldner BG, Maccaro PC, et al. A comparison of active compression-decompression cardiopulmonary resuscitation with standard cardiopulmonary resuscitation for cardiac arrests occurring in the hospital. *NEJM* 1993;329;1918–1921.

5 What's New, What's Different

1. State how the AHA classifies effectiveness of drugs.
2. Describe some of the changes that the AHA has made to selected algorithms.
3. List drug additions to the resuscitation protocols recommended by the AHA.

From Certification to Education

Changes in the ACLS course reflect a need to keep up with the new information available in the literature, but they also address the failings of the previous format. Many of the concerns and frustrations instructors and providers alike have felt with the previous ACLS format have been addressed. The course now utilizes an approach to teaching the management of cardiac arrhythmias, cardiac disease, and cardiac arrest that necessitates a wider knowledge of the drugs used and a keener understanding of what drug to use in what clinical setting. The teaching requires the participant to concentrate on the patient and on the patient's presentation rather than the rhythm on the monitor.

The method of instruction and the philosophy of the course has also changed. It is assumed that the participant is in the course because of a need for utilization of the skills and knowledge for patient resuscitation. With this premise and the understanding of adult education, the purpose of the course has changed. The need to "certify" participants often led to the course becoming a method of weeding out those participants not meeting the parameters to pass the skill stations and the exams. The new course concentrates on an educational orientation where evaluation in case-management scenarios allows the instructor to find areas of skill or knowledge deficiency and to pursue clarification and repeat instruction immediately. The emphasis is on ensuring that those participants who have a need of the knowledge and principles of ACLS will have it. The change to the case-management format instead of the lecture style finally allows us to address the frustration instructors and students felt during the mega code teaching stations. Many participants felt that valuable education was taking place mainly during that time and that one session was too little to achieve desired results.

The new course format may vary both in structure and in time allotment to allow for experience; however, participants must be able to master the core content of the course. The most important of the core content being the ability to assess and manage the first 10 minutes of an adult ventricular fibrillation cardiac arrest. The importance of early defibrillation is emphasized by this change.

Classification of Drugs

Drugs are not utilized in a routine scheme, but are classified as to their effectiveness based on studies and clinical results.

Class I drugs	those shown to be definitely effective
Class IIa drugs	those that are acceptable, probably effective
Class IIb drugs	those that are acceptable, possibly effective
Class III drugs	those that are not indicated and may be harmful

Use of these drugs requires not only an understanding of their pharmacology but also of their varying effect in different clinical settings. The best example of this is atropine. In symptomatic bradycardia atropine is a Class I drug. Knowledge of the possible side effects of atropine is important in its utilization and choice of dose, as higher doses may precipitate tachyarrhythmias and increased myocardial oxygen demand. Atropine is considered a Class III drug in patients with an acute anterior wall MI and third-degree heart block with ventricular escape beats. It is also Class III for use in patients with acute MI with Mobitz Type II second-degree block, as it fails to improve the atrioventricular (AV) block and it may speed up the sinus rate and actually worsen the block.[1] Clearly, administration of these medications not only requires knowledge of their classification in each clinical setting but also an understanding of the literature leading to the classification decision.

IVs, ETs, and Precordial Thump

Normal saline (NS) is the preferred intravenous (IV) solution for the cardiac arrest situation. It is most compatible with all medications and is without the poorer neurologic outcome that is associated with hyperglycemia. This also allows for volume expansion without changing the IV solution if indicated by clinical parameters or history.

Medications given down the endotracheal (ET) tube are given at 2 to 2.5 times the IV dose and *epinephrine, lidocaine,* and *atropine* may be administered via this route. The recommended dilution amount is 10 cc of normal saline or distilled water.[2,3]

The precordial thump is still included, but it is limited to the treatment of ventricular fibrillation (VF) or ventricular tachycardia (VT) when there is no pulse, no defibrillator immediately available, and a witnessed arrest. The precordial thump is not often successful and may lead to a deterioration of the rhythm.

Algorithms

The first algorithm is the universal algorithm for adult emergency cardiac care. The new emphasis is on early EMS or code team activation as soon as unresponsiveness is recognized. This allows for the earlier arrival of the capability to defibrillate in addition to all other components of ACLS. Throughout the algorithm, there is an emphasis on early defibrillation and early intervention with those modalities proven most effective being utilized frequently and to their maximum.

The pulseless electrical activity (PEA) algorithm replaces the electromechanical dissociation (EMD) algorithm. The EMD algorithm was awkward to teach and to utilize in a realistic clinical approach. Many cases of EMD were not truly EMD and led to much confusion. Often there was mechanical activity, but a clinical pulse was not detectable. The term *pulseless electrical activity* is more appropriate clinically. The algorithm again stresses the need to determine an underlying cause to be able to proceed with the most appropriate therapies. Included now is the recognition that PEA may have varied pulse rates, and further therapies may depend on that rate.

Wide-complex tachycardia of uncertain type fills in the gap of how to treat this group of patients while their specific rhythm is being debated. If the rate is >150 and the patient is unstable, cardioversion is recommended. If the patient is stable, lidocaine is considered a Class I agent for this rhythm (as is procainamide), but lidocaine remains the first drug of choice. Even though a Class I agent, procainamide is the third-line drug of choice due to its side effect of hypotension and to the length of time needed for administration. The second-line drug of choice in wide-complex tachycardia is adenosine even though it is a Class IIa agent. In addition to adenosine's rapid onset and lack of hypotensive effects, no clinical deteriorations have occurred even in administration during VT.

Two other new algorithms have been added and deal with the clinical presentation of acute MI and hypotension, shock, and pulmonary edema. Acute MI stresses early recognition and early treatment. The second algorithm addresses treatments of inadequate cardiac output due to a wide variety of etiologies and clinical presentation.

Changes in Doses of Old Drugs

Epinephrine doses have had the most variation and discussion and, after review of clinical trials at the National Conference on Cardiopulmonary Resuscitation and Emergency Cardiac Care in 1992,[4,5,6] it was determined there was no statistical difference in the survival rates with higher dosages of epinephrine compared with standard dosages. Therefore, it is still recommended that the initial dose of epinephrine be 1 mg IV. However, the new recommendation is to administer it every 3 to 5 minutes. The ET dose is 2 to 2.5 times that of the IV dose. High-dose epinephrine is neither recommended nor discouraged but can be considered for the second and subsequent doses as a Class IIb agent. Dose recommendations based on these trial reviews are consistent with the suggestion that asystole and PEA may have an increased survival with the high-dose regimen and that those patients over 65 do better with the standard dose.

Lidocaine is considered Class IIb for prophylaxis in acute MI and is not routinely recommended. For other indications, the initial bolus of 1 to 1.5 mg/kg is recommended with subsequent doses of 0.5 to 1.5 mg/kg to a total of 3 mg/kg. The higher dose range is suggested for cardiac arrest and the lower for less acute situations, keeping in mind the narrow therapeutic range and possible side effects especially in those patients with the highest potential for toxicity. For example, in VF after appropriate defibrillation and epinephrine administration, lidocaine 1.5 mg/kg IV is administered, in 3 to 5 minutes another 1.5 mg/kg IV may be administered (assuming appropriate defibrillation and epinephrine administration). If defibrillation is successful after the first bolus, a subsequent bolus of 0.5 mg/kg may be given to a total of 2 mg/kg unless arrhythmias continue.

Procainamide is now given as an infusion of 20 mg/min (may be 30 mg/min in critical situations) with the same end point of resolution of the arrhythmia, widening of the QRS > 50%, or hypotension. The total dose is now 17 mg/kg instead of 1 gm.

Atropine is now given to a total of 0.04 mg/kg. At this time, there is no mg/kg suggested for each dose, the range is still 0.5 to 1 mg. It is important when selecting a dosage in this range to remember that lower doses may be associated with paradoxical slowing of the heart rate and higher doses may be associated with tachyarrhythmias. The dose chosen should be appropriate to the patient's size and clinical condition.

Drug Deletions and Additions

Sodium bicarbonate, although not eliminated, has certainly been decreased in its importance. In its place is the increased emphasis on adequate ventilation and early reversal of the arrest rhythm. Sodium bicarbonate is indicated in some clinical situations such as hyperkalemia, known metabolic acidosis, phenobarbital, and tricyclic overdoses. Here, again, is an emphasis on the clinical history and the tailoring of treatment to the patient. For example, if an arrest victim is a renal dialysis patient, earlier consideration will be given to the use of sodium bicarbonate as a drug of choice in cardiac arrest.

Verapamil usage is limited to the treatment of narrow-complex paroxysmal supraventricular tachycardia (PSVT) and only as a second-line drug after adenosine. It is also utilized for rate control in atrial fibrillation.

Indicated uses for isoproterenol are significantly less. It is classified as a Class IIb drug at low doses and as a Class III drug at higher doses. Isoproterenol is a Class IIa drug in refractory torsades de pointes and in symptomatic bradycardia in the denervated hearts of transplant patients.

Adenosine is considered the first-line drug for PSVT as it has fewer side effects than verapamil. It is considered second-line in the treatment of wide QRS tachycardia of unknown etiology (lidocaine and procainamide are the first-line drugs) since it has not been shown to be detrimental in VT and has been successful in converting this rhythm.[7,8,9] It is important to remember that adenosine must be used with caution in patients taking dipyridamole. The effects of adenosine may be more pronounced and last longer in these patients. A smaller dose (1 mg to start) or another drug should be utilized.[10] In those patients taking theophylline or other methylxanthines, larger doses may be required due to receptor site competition. Carbamazepine also blocks the receptor sites for adenosine and thus may cause it to be less effective. In addition, carbamazepine also has been reported to increase the degree of heart block produced by other agents and, as a primary effect of adenosine is to slow conduction at the AV node, higher degrees of blockade may occur when these drugs are used together.[11]

Magnesium is considered the drug of choice in torsades de pointes. Although several studies suggest routine use of magnesium in acute MIs, recent literature has not proven it to be of benefit.[12,13] Magnesium is also recommended for those patients felt to be deficient in magnesium levels and may be also useful for those patients for whom thrombolysis is not an option.[14]

More Recent Articles

New findings from the ISIS–4 study provides important information to be included in an ACLS course regarding the treatment of acute MIs. It is a large study including over 50,000 patients that bears review by those instructors charged with the responsibility of teaching cardiac care providers. Many controversies have been addressed in the study and the results of that study should be included when instructing ACLS. One important change as a result of these studies will be the increased use of angiotensin converting enzyme (ACE) inhibitors in acute MIs due to the drug's apparent ability to cause a reduced mortality, especially with high-risk patients.[15]

Another recent study using aminophylline for the treatment of bradyasystolic cardiac arrest bears attention. Although the number of patients studied was small (15 patients), the results were interesting both from a physiologic point of view and as a potential means of treating asystole. Aminophylline 250 mg IV was administered to patients in arrest with asystole or severe bradyarrhythmia (< 30 bpm) who had not responded to atropine (≥ 2 mg) and epinephrine (≥ 2 mg). Of the 15 patients, 11 developed a rhythm after injection of aminophylline. However, only one patient was finally discharged from the hospital without brain damage.[15]

Psychological Features of Resuscitation

Although only a short section in the new guidelines, this topic is important in its inclusion not only for its importance in how to relate to the family but in its acceptance of the fact that there are many components of the resuscitation that are stressful not only to the family but to the health-care provider as well. We have all recognized with experience that it is important to know what to say to a family to inform them of a death as well as know what to tell them in anticipation of their questions and fears. Included are recommendations on how to help the family as well as recommendations on code debriefing for health-care providers (see Tables 5.1 and 5.2).

■ **Table 5.1**   Conveying News of a Sudden Death to Family Members

Call the family if they have not been notified. Explain that their loved one has been admitted to the emergency department and that the situation is serious. Survivors should not be told of the death over the telephone.

Obtain as much information as possible about the patient and the circumstances surrounding the death. Carefully go over the events as they happened in the emergency department.

Ask someone to take family members to a private area. Walk in, introduce yourself, and sit down. Address the closest relative.

Briefly describe the circumstances leading to the death. Go over the sequence of events in the emergency department. Avoid euphemisms such as "he's passed on," "she's no longer with us," or "he's left us." Instead, use the words "death," "dying," or "dead."

Allow time for the shock to be absorbed. Make eye contact, touch, and share. Convey your feelings with a phrase such as "You have my (our) sincere sympathy" rather than "I (we) am sorry."

Allow as much time as necessary for questions and discussion. Go over the events several times to make sure everything is understood and to facilitate further questions.

Allow the family the opportunity to see their relative. If equipment is still connected, let the family know.

Know in advance what happens next and who will sign the death certificate. Physicians may impose burdens on staff and family if they fail to understand policies about death certification and disposition of the body. Know the answers to these questions before meeting the family.

Enlist the aid of a social worker or the clergy if not already present.

Offer to contact the patient's attending or family physician and to be available if there are further questions. Arrange for follow-up and continued support during the grieving period.

Reproduced with permission. CPR Issue. JAMA, October 28, 1992. © American Heart Association.

Summary

The new ACLS guidelines emphasize education of the community at large and medical personnel of the need for early recognition and treatment. The emphasis is in those situations where early recognition and intervention will make a difference in morbidity and mortality.

■ **Table 5.2**   **Recommendations for Critical Incident Debriefing**

The debriefing should occur as soon as possible after the event, with all team members present.
Call the group together, preferably in the resuscitation room. State that you want to have a "code debriefing."
Review the events and conduct of the code. Include the contributory pathophysiology leading to the code, the decision tree followed, and any variations.
Analyze the things that were done wrong and especially the things that were done right. Allow free discussion.
Ask for recommendations/suggestions for future resuscitative attempts.
All team members should share their feelings, anxieties, anger, and possible guilt.
Team members unable to attend the debriefing should be informed of the process followed, the discussion generated, and the recommendations made.
The team leader should encourage team members to contact him or her if questions arise later.

Reproduced with permission. CPR Issue. JAMA, October 28, 1992. © American Heart Association.

The new ACLS guidelines are reflective of this awareness of the need to base our treatment on clinical grounds. Treatment choices are expected to be made on a clinical basis, *not* on a rote algorithm. This will require more work on the part of instructors to produce a course that is clinically based with variations not on rhythm but on clinical presentation. Hopefully, this will reflect on the actual management of the cardiac arrest with more emphasis placed on patient history of present illness and on the patient's past medical history.

Many controversies have been clarified; however, many new ones have surfaced creating the need for continued review of the literature for information regarding results of good studies on which to base decision making for the treatment of patients. The guidelines are written with enough variation in treatment options to encourage the utilization of new treatments based on changes in the literature, but the clinician bears the responsibility of knowledge of that literature prior to teaching and to treatment of the patient in a cardiac arrest situation. The guidelines can only be utilized appropriately by those who are knowledgeable of the information on which they are based.

References

1. Rapaport E, Fuster V, Reeves TJ, et al. Guidelines for the early management of patients with acute myocardial infarction: A report of the American College of Cardiology/American Heart Association Task Force on Assessment of Diagnostic and Therapeutic Cardiovascular Procedures. *J Am Coll Cardiol* 1990;16:249–292.

2. Aitkenhead AR. Drug administration during CPR; what route? *Resuscitation* 1991;22:191–195.

3. Hahnel JH, Lindner KH, Schurmann C, et al. Plasma lidocaine levels and PaO_2 with endobronchial administration: Dilution with normal saline or distilled water? *Ann Emerg Med* 1990;19:1314–1317.

4. Lindner KH, Ahnefeld FW, Prengel A. Comparison of standard and high-dose adrenaline in the resuscitation of asystole and electromechanical dissociation. *Acta Anaesthesiol Scand* 1991;35:253–256.

5. Steill IG, Hebert PC, Weitzman BN, et al. A study of high-dose epinephrine in human CPR. *Ann Emerg Med* 1992;21:606. Abstract.

6. Callaham M, Madsen CD, Barton CW, et al. A randomized clinical trial of high-dose epinephrine and norepinephrine versus standard-dose epinephrine in prehospital cardiac arrest. *Ann Emerg Med* 1992;21:606–607. Abstract.

7. Rankin AC, Oldroyd KG, Chong E, et al. Value and limitations of adenosine in the diagnosis and treatment of narrow and broad complex tachycardias. *Br Heart J* 1989;62:195–302.

8. Griffith MJ, Linker NJ, Ward DE, et al. Adenosine in the diagnosis of broad complex tachycardia. *Lancet* 1988;1(8587):672–675.

9. Sharma AD, Klein GJ, Yee Y. Intravenous adenosine triphosphate during wide QRS complex tachycardia: Safety, therapeutic efficacy, and diagnostic utility. *Am J Med* 1990;88:337–343.

10. Freilich A, Tepper D. Adenosine and its cardiovascular effects. *Am Heart J* 1992;123:1324–1328.

11. Kasarskis EJ, Kuo CS, Berger R, et al. Carbamazepine induced cardiac dysfunction. *Arch Intern Med* 1992;152(1):186–191.

12. ISIS Collaborative Group. ISIS–4: Randomized study of intravenous magnesium in over 50,000 patients with suspected acute myocardial infarction. *Circulation* 1993;88(4, pt 2):1–292. Abstract.

13. Epstein SE. Highlights of the 65th scientific sessions of the American Heart Association. *J Myocard Isch* 1994;6(2):9–13.

14. Shechter M, Hod H, Kaplinsky E, et al. Magnesium as alternate therapy in acute myocardial infarction patients unsuited for thrombolysis. *Circulation* 1993;88(4, pt 2):1–395. Abstract.

15. Viskin S, Belhassen B, Roth A, et al. Aminophylline for bradysystolic cardiac arrest refractory to atropine and epinephrine. *Ann Intern Med* 1993; 118:279–281.

6 Airway Management: The Critical First Step

Objectives

1. Describe the changes in recommended ventilation procedures and know the approach to proper airway management.
2. State the appropriate use of the bag-valve-mask.
3. Be able to identify the indications for ET intubation.

Basic Airway Management

Airway management is an integral part of both the ACLS program and basic CPR curriculum. Due to its importance in resuscitation its occasional review and clarification is essential. The "A" in "ABCs" is not emphasized without reason. Without an adequate airway, all of your other efforts on the patient's behalf are wasted. A patient's airway may be compromised without dramatic outward signs. Without a gag reflex, the patient's tongue won't clear the airway. In all cases, a questionable airway must be suspected and, if found, must be dealt with in a speedy and efficient manner. The management techniques utilized will depend on the situation and skills of the health care provider. Assessing your airway management skills will be performed either during the case-based teaching stations or in a separate airway management skills station.

There are numerous techniques available to alleviate airway compromise. A thorough knowledge of them will enable the ACLS/CPR provider to fit the solution to the problem and also have some alternative methods available in case the initial method doesn't accomplish the job. In order to fit the solution to the problem, the health care provider must know the technique and its indications. This chapter will attempt to present some of these techniques with hints for their appropriate use.

Manual Methods

Manual methods of airway management are primarily used for a tongue obstruction. They are of little value in management of a patient with a foreign-body obstruction of the airway. These foreign-body obstructions are managed by obstructed airway maneuvers and/or suctioning. The anatomy of the oropharynx is such that an unconscious, supine person will quickly lose airway patency due to the tongue falling back in the posterior oropharynx. Basic airway management is directed toward preventing this occurrence or alleviating the problem if it has occurred. Do not forget to mention this during the mega code/case-based teaching station and/or in the airway station.

Head Tilt/Neck Lift

The head tilt/neck lift has been shown to be less effective than the head tilt/chin lift method in clearing the tongue from the posterior oropharynx.[1,2] It is also extremely dangerous in the cervical (C)-spine injured patient and is **no longer taught in AHA courses**.

Infants' necks should not be placed in a hyperextended position. They have soft cartilage rings in their tracheas, which do not tolerate the squeezing imparted by such a position and can, in fact, collapse and obstruct a previously clear airway. The infant's large occiput tends to place him or her in a sniffing position. A gentle lift of the chin is usually all that is required to give the infant a good airway.

Head Tilt/Chin Lift

The head tilt/chin lift is the preferred method of opening an airway that may be blocked by the patient's tongue. The basic concept is to elevate the jaw causing the tongue to be pulled forward/anterior. This works because the tongue is anchored at the hyoid bone, which is embedded in the soft tissue of the lower jaw.

Jaw Thrust

The jaw thrust is performed by placing the fingers at the angle of the jaw (with your thumbs on the cheekbones for stabilization), as you are moving the lower jaw forward. With this method, the tongue is moved out of the oral pharynx area. This technique causes no manipulation of the C-spine so this is the preferred technique for all trauma patients.

This technique requires manual dexterity and practice to become fully comfortable with the procedure. However, maintaining this awkward position for extended periods of time can cause muscle cramps even in well-trained individuals.

Sniffing Position

If you have witnessed any patient in acute respiratory distress, you will note that the patient tends to project his head forward while at the same time tilting it back. This is called the *sniffing* position. Patients in respiratory distress tend to assume this position because it gives them the best airway possible. Note that if a patient is supine in bed, the position can't be achieved by placing a towel under the shoulders. It must be obtained by placing some padding under the *head*. It is also the most advantageous position to place the patient in order to pass an ET tube.

Basic Airway Devices

Oropharyngeal Airway

The oropharyngeal airway (OPA) (Figure 6.1) is the most basic airway management tool. Although it is relatively safe and efficient, it does have potential drawbacks and limitations. The first of these is the assumption on some practitioners' part that the device is a guaranteed airway. Its *only* purpose is to hold the tongue out of the way so you do not have to manually hold the head tilt/chin lift or jaw thrust. It is *not* a de-

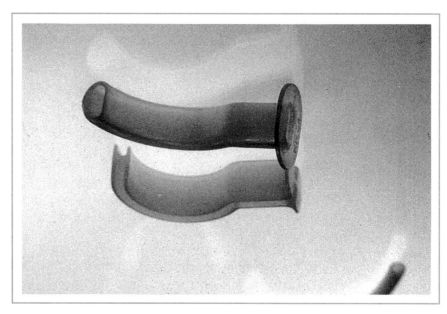

■ **Figure 6.1**   Oropharyngeal airway (OPA).

finitive airway. Patients can and do vomit through it. The OPA should only be placed in patients who **do not** have an intact gag reflex.

Sizing of airways is of critical importance. In adults, too small an airway may be "eaten" by the patient and has the potential to obstruct the airway. In the child, too large an airway may damage the posterior oropharynx or obstruct the airway. Sizing is done by measuring the distance from the lips to angle of the jaw or ear lobe. This step should not be skipped, as the results can be catastrophic.

Placement is the last area where hazardous situations can occur. Most of us were taught to place the airway in the patient's mouth upside down with the curved area toward the patient's tongue and then taught to rotate the device into place. It has been recognized that early rotation and aggressive placement can force the tongue *down* and *obstruct the airway*.[3,4] Currently, students are being taught to rotate the OPA early, but *only halfway,* (so it faces either cheek), and do most of the insertion in this position. Insertion of the airway sideways is also a viable and preferred method of placement. If you have picked the appropriate sized airway, it will literally rotate itself into position when it contacts the posterior oropharynx. Do not try to hurry it along by rotating it early. The risk of a forced tongue obstruction is too great.

During your ACLS course, you may be exposed to the OPA and should become familiar with its uses and limitations. You will also learn during the course that you can ventilate a person without an OPA.

Nasopharyngeal Airway

The nasopharyngeal airway (NPA) (Figure 6.2) is another device gaining in popularity since it does have distinct advantages in some common emergency situations. Those patients who need a basic airway and yet will not tolerate an OPA are the prime candidates for the NPA. Some examples of such patients are those presenting with a stroke, drug ingestion, alcohol overdose, head injury, or a clenched jaw. They may all need assistance with airway maintenance, yet do not require endotracheal intubation and will not tolerate an oropharyngeal airway. These sonorous patients are usually excellent candidates for an NPA, which has the significant advantage of *not* stimulating a gag reflex in semiconscious patients. When presented with this type of patient during your

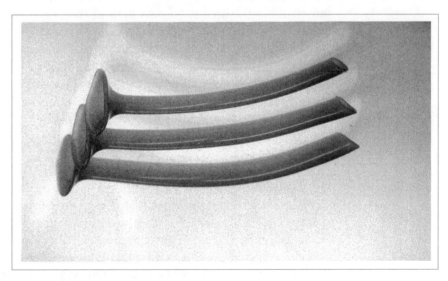

■ **Figure 6.2**   Nasopharyngeal airway (NPA).

mega code/case-based teaching station, it would be wise to inform the instructor that you would place an NPA into the patient.

It can be measured in much the same way as the OPA, from the nose to the angle of the jaw or earlobe. They now come in internal diameter sizes, much the same as an ET tube, and range in size from 6.0 mm to 9.0 mm with the length of the tube varying with the internal diameter. Many find the 6.0 mm to 8.0 mm airways the most useful and this size range can be used for the small, medium, and large adult. Be very cautious about using too long an airway as it can direct your ventilations into the esophagus causing hypoventilation and death or, if in the trachea, possibly laryngospasm (which may often prove fatal).[4] Lubrication of the device will aid with placement and, along with careful insertion, may reduce trauma to the tubernates.

The device is placed in either nostril and is inserted at a right angle to the face, **not** in an upward direction. Pushing the tip of the nose up with your finger while inserting the airway will tend to keep the airway directed at a 90° angle. Therefore, the airway is directed toward the posterior nasopharynx. A gentle back-and-forth rotation of the airway may aid insertion. When the flared end is about an inch from the nares, the airway will usually stop moving. It stops because the distal end is against the back of the tongue. The next step is to simply lift the jaw to allow the airway to pass behind the posterior tongue. This airway usually does not stimulate the gag reflex after insertion and is exceptionally well tolerated by the semiconscious individual. These airways should be soft and compliant to minimize any trauma and should be considered in any "in between" airway management problem.

Ventilation

General Concepts

Aggressive ventilation of the *nonbreathing* patient has rarely injured someone with the notable exception of patients with chronic obstructive pulmonary disease. With these patients, there is always the risk of causing a pneumothorax with excessive ventilation pressures (assume that respiratory drive is not an issue here as you are already engaged in ventilating the patient).

However, faster rates of ventilation are not precluded up to the limits allowed by the patient's diseased respiratory system. For most patients undergoing CPR, ventilation rates of once every second or third compression should prove adequate. With these ventilation rates, typical blood gas results in cardiac arrest are PaO_2 readings in the range of 300 to 400, pH of approximately 7.25, and $PaCO_2$ readings in the range of 25 to 27. Ventilating at rates faster than this result in very high O_2 concentrations (500+), but have the problem of reducing CO_2 to levels around ±18, which can be detrimental to the patient's neurologic status.

With these facts in mind, **always** ventilate early and aggressively for any patient who needs it.

Two Key Points

1. If you think the patient will have to be ventilated in the next half hour, ventilate the patient now.
2. If the patient tolerates being hand ventilated with a bag-valve-mask, then continue to ventilate.

In an ACLS course setting you may have to ask your instructor what type of condition your patient has when presented with a specific case scenario.

Use in Breathing Patients

Ventilation with a bag-valve-mask (BVM) or demand valve can usually be tolerated by some conscious patients in respiratory distress; classically, pulmonary edema. If the patient does not tolerate the ventilation, then high-flow O_2 by mask should be continued. A close watch must be kept on this patient as CO_2 build-up (CO_2 narcosis) can stop the patient's respirations. This change may be so subtle as to not be immediately recognized by the caregiver. Watch the patient. A blind nasotracheal tube will probably have to be placed if the patient's respirations become depressed so that the ventilations need to be assisted.

Maintaining ventilations in children is especially important as their problems often revolve around ventilation/respiration defects. A child who normally has respirations of about 20/min does not tolerate respirations of 10/ min for very long.

Techniques

Mouth to Mask Mouth-to-mask techniques became a procedure of choice with the possibility of contracting a communicable disease from a patient. They are simple to use and can provide very good tidal volumes to the hypoxic patient. Since utilization of a BVM is awkward and requires much repetition to maintain one's skill level, poor performance has been recognized using this device unless well trained. For this reason, some hospitals have been replacing the BVM units on the floors with pocket masks. Anesthesia or respiratory personnel can subsequently bring the BVM with them when responding to an emergency.

The use of a mouth-to-mask device requires an excellent mask seal for maximum effectiveness. The use of a one-way valve for the health care provider is strongly recommended. The best way to utilize this device appears to start by positioning yourself at the head of the patient,[5] producing a mask seal by either encircling the mask with the index finger and thumb of each hand or using the thumbs in a spreading motion over the top of the mask to hold a good mask seal. The remaining fingers then go under the lower jaw and the hands are gently squeezed to ensure the mask seal. At the same time, the jaw is lifted with the hands to clear the tongue. If an OPA or NPA tube is available, it can be utilized to maintain a patent airway. This device can, with care, be used on the traumatized patient in the same way that the trauma airway is utilized.

When this device is used without supplemental oxygen, the O_2 delivered is less than that of room air ($\pm 16\%$). An oxygen inlet is, therefore, necessary. As soon as possible, the device should be connected to high-flow O_2, (15 L/min) and ventilations continued. The O_2 concentrations received by the patient will approach 50%, which will greatly assist the hypoxic patient.[6]

Manually Triggered Oxygen-Powered Breathing Devices (Demand Valves) These devices supply oxygen to the patient when a lever is pulled or a button pushed. There is nothing to squeeze and the operator can spend more effort in maintaining a good mask seal. It was used for a number of years with flow rates of up to 100 L/min. Gastric distension caused by excessive ventilation and/or poor airway maintenance has been a major problem with this device and is not without sequelae for the patient. Elevation of the diaphragm can and does occur and will impede airflow to the lungs and can also lead to vomiting, making airway management much more complicated, and could lead to aspiration.

For these reasons, the AHA has recommended[3] that manually triggered, oxygen-powered breathing devices

1. Be limited to a constant flow rate of less than 40 L/min O_2
2. Have an inspiratory relief valve that opens at approximately 60 cm H_2O
3. Vent any remaining volume to the atmosphere or cease gas flow
4. Have an audible alarm that sounds whenever the relief valve pressure is exceeded to alert the health care provider that the patient is requiring high inflation pressures
5. Have satisfactory operation under common environmental conditions/temperatures
6. Have a demand flow system that does not impose additional work

Even after listing the preceding problems, however, the device does have important uses. The demand valve can also supply O_2 on demand to the breathing patient or be manually overridden to supply an extra volume to the compromised patient. With the present less than 40 L/min O_2 flow-rate limitations, these devices may be recommended over BVMs for ventilation of the *non*intubated patient as the problems of gastric distension currently encountered may not be present.

The demand valve may not be a good choice for use with ET tubes. When a tube is in place, a BVM with supplemental O_2 is preferred for its "feel" and simplicity of use.[7] Also, this device is designed for adults and can cause injury to the pediatric population.

Bag-Valve-Mask   The BVM (Figure 6.3) is the original manually powered breathing device. Properly used, it is safe, effective, and allows a considerable amount of feedback to allow the emergency health care responder to judge the effectiveness of the ventilation efforts.

In practice, it is significantly more difficult to use than would seem at first glimpse. It takes extensive practice to become and stay proficient in the use of this device. If this is not possible, ventilations should take place utilizing a mouth-to-mouth device with supplemen-

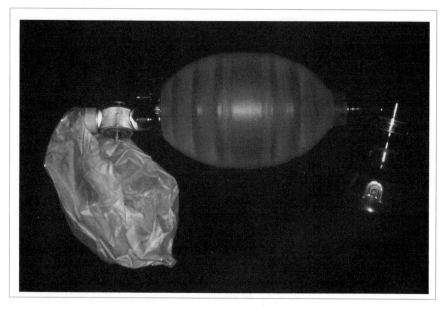

Figure 6.3   Bag-valve-mask (BVM).

tal oxygen until an ET tube can be placed.[3] Just placing the mask on the face and squeezing the bag may have the appearance of assisting the patient, but it does little more than give the operator some hand exercise and is all the worse for the false sense of security it gives the rescuer. It is best if two people can operate the BVM.[8] During all ACLS courses, you should spend an adequate amount of practice time to become comfortable with the proper use of the BVM. However, this is impractical in most situations. To use the device properly,

1. An oral airway should be placed (although not always necessary).
2. An excellent mask seal must be obtained and be able to be held with only one hand (though still difficult, this is made easier with some of the new mask designs).
3. Proper head tilt (airway) must be maintained (*only* if C-spine compromise is not a consideration).
4. Good ventilation must be obtained by squeezing the bag properly.

Problems may emerge in maintaining head tilt/mask seal and actually getting adequate ventilation from the bag when held in one hand.

Practice using the equipment will be required to avoid this potential complication.

Head Tilt, Airway and Mask Seal

While relatively easy to demonstrate initially, holding the position while attempting to maintain a mask seal can be difficult. To seat the mask, one must place the index finger and thumb around the mask near the connector, with the remaining fingers going under the jaw to squeeze the mask onto the face. The arm is then used to gain and maintain head tilt while ventilation continues with the other.

When ventilation continues for long periods of time and/or while moving, problems in maintaining this position can and do occur rapidly. What makes this more ominous is that these problems develop somewhat gradually and the operator may not recognize them. The same difficulties can also occur with the demand valve, but with a BVM there is an advantage.

Ventilation

This is an area where a good many health care providers fail to achieve acceptable results. Most ventilating bags are advertised as delivering 1200 cc to 1600 cc of volume. These volumes can usually be achieved only by the concerted use of both hands. If you only have one hand available for ventilation, the other being tied up holding the mask and head tilt, achieving good results is exceedingly difficult. In order to successfully ventilate the patient, the entire bag must be rolled into the hand using the bed, your leg or hip, or even the patient's head to push the bag against to achieve the volumes necessary for adequate ventilation. The other option, as stated earlier, is to have one person hold the mask seal while the other squeezes the bag using both hands. In either case, the proper ventilation volumes must be maintained at acceptable levels, or patient care suffers. It is a skill that must be maintained with practice.

The lung compliance that the operator feels when ventilating the patient will change due to increased resistance. This should signal the operator to change something in his or her technique to achieve the desired results. Although ventilating a manikin is difficult and differs in some ways from actual application, it will give a reasonable simulation of the difficulties in using the technique and is a worthwhile skill to review. If you ventilate patients infrequently, you should practice more often, not less. The skill deteriorates *rapidly* over time.

This review of basic airway techniques will not take the place of hands-on instruction and practice during case-based teaching stations in the ACLS course. We urge you to keep your skills up to par for the best interest of your patient who depends on your skills for survival. This is best done on a regular basis and not only when you are attending an ACLS course. The next section of this chapter will review advanced airway techniques and their application.

Advanced Airway Management

Endotracheal Intubation

Visualized Oral Endotracheal Intubation

Endotracheal intubation remains the gold standard for airway management and is one of the requirements for successful completion of the ACLS course. Endotracheal intubation utilizes a laryngoscope of varying designs and materials or a fiberoptic device to enable visualization of the vocal cords by movement of those anatomic structures that impeded vision of the vocal cords. A hollow plastic tube fitted with an inflatable cuff is then passed slightly beyond the cords and the cuff inflated to obtain a guaranteed airway (Figure 6.4). This cuff is necessary because the adult trachea is larger below the cords than above it.

Most providers have found the crossed-finger technique to be the most satisfactory and safe method to open the mouth. If the patient suddenly decides to bite down, there is a tendency for your fingers to snap out of the mouth rather than become engaged by the patient's teeth.

The standard ET tube cuff holds 10 cc of air. If, however, you are able to fill the standard cuff with 10 cc of air, you probably could have gone at least one-half tube size larger. Tubes come in various sizes with the internal diameter mark indicating the size in millimeters (e.g., 7.0 mm, 7.5 mm, 8.0 mm, and larger). The length of each tube is also marked by centimeters. For most adults, the normal length for place-

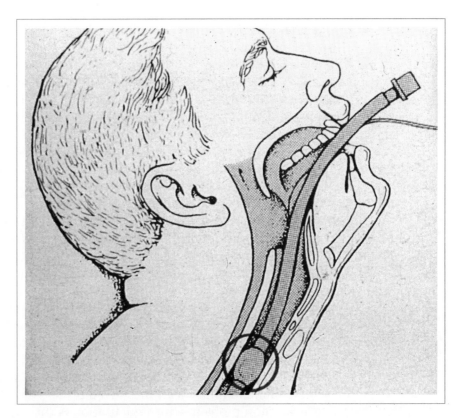

■ **Figure 6.4**   **Visualized oral endotracheal intubation.**

ment of the tube will be found at the 20 cm to 22 cm mark by measuring against the front teeth. Some of the newer tubes use a high-volume/low-pressure cuff, which may take more than the standard 10 cc of air. They have the advantage of using less pressure to achieve an adequate seal. *Know your equipment!* Spend some extra time familiarizing yourself with the equipment and manikin at the airway station and/or the case-based teaching station.

The intubation process should not be rushed and the proper equipment needs to be ready prior to initiating an intubation attempt. The patient is always ventilated by other means prior to ET intubation. When you have your equipment ready and the patient has been ventilated, the intubation attempt can then proceed. Since some ACLS airway manikins are in better condition than others, consider practicing intubation on each one to perfect your technique.

The laryngoscope is slid into the mouth and the tongue swept left. **DO NOT USE ANY PRYING MOTION ON THE HANDLE AND BY NO MEANS USE THE TEETH AS A FULCRUM.** The laryngoscope is a left-handed instrument whether you are left- or right-handed. The epiglottis is visualized and, if using a curved blade, it is lifted indirectly by utilizing gentle force in the direction the handle is pointing. The curved blade should be in the vallecula. If you are using a straight blade, it is dipped down and the epiglottis is lifted directly. Some practitioners prefer the curved blade because there is less chance of causing bradycardia by stimulating the vagus nerve through manipulation of the epiglottis. Others prefer a straight blade because they feel that it gives them better control. In any case, if you are unsuccessful with one type of blade, change blades, which often proves effective. Some anatomic shapes seem to adapt better to one shape than the other. In trauma with in-line stabilization of the neck, the straight blade seems to afford better visualization. In pediatrics, you are dealing with a slightly different anatomy with the larynx being more anterior and superior than in the adult. The curved blade will tend to have you aiming for the ceiling. In addition, the infant vallecula is smaller and may be more prone to injury with the curved blade.

A common problem with visualization is that the practitioner, in an attempt to visualize the cords, almost tries to "climb into the patient's mouth." In order to improve your visualization, try moving back. It tends to keep things in perspective and may help you see the anatomy better.

The most common error in technique is utilizing the laryngoscope like a claw hammer pulling out nails. Leveraging off the teeth not only is extremely harmful but obstructs your view of the anatomy. In training students, a "cock-up" wrist fracture splint works well to keep the student from bending his or her wrist thereby lessening the tendency to lever off the teeth.

After visualization of the vocal cords, the tube is passed until the cuff on the tube is just distal to the cords. If you do not see the cords, don't pass the tube. There are techniques that don't require cord visualization. This is not one of them. Having seen the cords, don't pass the tube too far. Right mainstem bronchus intubation can cause hypoventilation and collapse of the left lung. Right mainstem intubation can and does occur even after a proper intubation. Through any number of scenarios, the tube gets advanced during the transportation process. **Reassess . . . reassess . . . reassess!**

If the attempt is not successful, get out of the patient's face and ventilate him or her with other means. Holding your breath can give you an idea of the time limit that exists that will cause the patient distress. When you are uncomfortable, you know the patient is becoming more hypoxic.

Since this procedure is not well tolerated by the awake patient, the patient is usually unresponsive although necessity sometimes dictates that the patient will be marginally responsive when the procedure takes place. If this is the situation, you may want to consider an alternative method of ventilation.

Complications

The following are complications that can be encountered when performing ET intubation:

* Hypoxemia from prolonged intubation attempts
* Right mainstem intubation
* Loose or broken teeth
* Esophageal intubation
* Trauma to the airway
* Vomiting leading to aspiration
* Avulsion of the vocal cords
* In trauma patients, there is the potential to convert a C-spine injury without neurologic deficit to a C-spine injury with neurologic deficit

Nasotracheal Intubation

Sometimes referred to as blind nasotracheal intubation, this method is being used more frequently with patients who are marginally conscious when intubation is necessitated. It is most useful in pulmonary edema patients, drug overdoses, and selected trauma patients. It is primarily used for conscious patients who need ventilatory assistance. Placing the tube is much like rolling the dice—very difficult since the tube is not visualized and placement is as dependent on luck as on skill. There is also a problem with bleeding as the posterior tubernates tend to be scraped during passage of the tube. The technique is explained to the patient, if awake, and a well-lubricated tube is passed through one of the nares to the posterior oropharynx where it is slid into the trachea with a gentle movement as the patient inhales. The patient may often be sitting up during this procedure and, if the head is tilted forward during the process (chin to chest), sometimes the tube is advanced more easily.

A modification of the classic technique can be utilized which addresses some of the following problems:

- The patient is assumed to be on high-flow oxygen, that appropriate exams have been accomplished, and that other remediation techniques are in progress.
- Neo-synephrine is instilled in both nostrils, either by spray or dropper. You may need to be generous in dosage to obtain maximum result. The oxygen mask is then replaced during further preparations.
- The ET tube is well-lubricated with a water-soluble jell. Sizes 7 mm to 8 mm will usually be appropriate for most patients.

The critical aspect of the procedure is as follows: A 10 Fr. suction catheter is obtained and the plastic "whistle" control tip is removed and discarded. The tubing itself is then placed over the metal tube of a Cetacaine spray bottle. The distal end of this tube is then advanced through the nares until maximum depth is obtained. The Cetacaine is then discharged deeply into the patient's posterior oropharynx and upper respiratory areas. The tube is withdrawn while continuing to spray and the process is repeated in the other nare. It is common for the patient to cough at this point if enough Cetacaine has been utilized.

The ET tube is then smoothly inserted in whichever nare is felt to have the greater diameter. If the tip of the nose is gently pushed upward, this part of the process tends to go more smoothly.

The tube is advanced while listening for increasing breath sounds at the proximal end. Cricoid pressure (Sellick maneuver), flexing the patient's head forward, and gently rotating the tube can assist the practitioner to successfully place the tube. The tube is assumed to be properly placed when misting occurs and frank respiration occurs through the tube. The cuff is inflated and the tube secured after confirmation of placement is assured by auscultation, radiography, and capnometry.

Situational Modifications

The Stylet

The stylet can be a powerful ally in intubating (oral intubation only) a difficult patient by providing a more extreme bend in the tube and maintaining this rigidity throughout the intubation (Figure 6.5). However, it can cause extreme damage if used incorrectly. Remember to keep the end of the stylet *at least* ½ inch back from the end of the tube prior to insertion. **Be careful** during removal of all stylets as they have been known to extubate patients if removed too rapidly.

Anchoring the Endotracheal Tube

There are a number of commercially available devices for maintaining ET tubes in place and the efficacy may vary from patient to patient. The standard umbilical tape works well in most circumstances, but it has a tendency to slip when wet and may also knot at the adapter site. What may also work is IV tubing. The plastic against plastic works very well and can hold even when wet. Additionally, it has some "give" in it that helps prevent breaking when stretched.

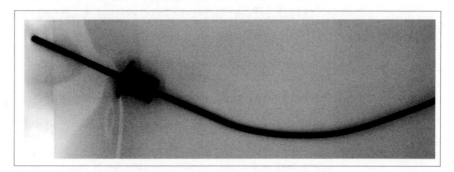

■ **Figure 6.5**   Stylet.

Transtracheal Catheter Ventilation

There are instances, while rare, where an airway obstruction of a patient is not relieved by the methods already discussed, and there may be a need to perform a needle cricothyrotomy. In these situations, this will be performed using a transtracheal catheter ventilation procedure.

One of the advantages of this method of airway control is that the landmarks are easily accessible and a needle can be inserted directly through the skin into the trachea. The needle is inserted caudally while maintaining negative pressure on the syringe. Once the catheter is inserted correctly (you should note no obvious blood in the syringe), the needle is then removed and oxygen connecting tubing from a 40 psi to 50 psi is attached for ventilation. The ventilation ratio (in seconds) of inflation to deflation is 1:4. It should also be noted that a gradual increase in the $PaCO_2$ may occur after 30 min to 45 min of ventilating a patient with this method.

Advantages to this procedure include

- No surgical procedures required
- Ease of access
- Minimal equipment
- Ease of insertion
- Minimal educational requirements

Combination Esophageal-Tracheal Tube and Pharyngotracheal Lumen Airway

The esophageal-tracheal (ETC) tube and pharyngotracheal lumen (PTL) airway are very similar in structure in that both are double-lumen devices that are inserted blindly into the esophagus. During your ACLS course case-based teaching stations, you may be asked by the instructor to either describe the advantages/disadvantages of these devices or to actually utilize them in the case with which you have been presented.

After an appropriate assessment of proper placement has been made, the patient is ventilated through the appropriate opening. The primary reasons for the development of these devices were to replace the deficiencies found in effecting a proper face seal as well as the inadvertent tracheal intubation that have occurred with the EOA/EGTA. Recent studies indicate that an inadequate seal with the pharyngeal balloon has been noted with the PTL airway as well.

In addition, there have been no comparative studies of the effectiveness of the PTL and basic airway techniques. The complication rates for both the ETC and PTL are low; however, further studies are required before the widespread endorsement of these airways can be granted.

Summary

Airway management is a critical component of all codes. The ACLS provider course will place major emphasis on airway control and ventilation. This will be accomplished during the case-based teaching stations. In some courses, the ACLS faculty may require the standard airway management skills station if they feel more practice time is required to master the techniques. Plan to spend extra time in this station if you feel you are not comfortable with the psychomotor skills necessary to demonstrate appropriate airway techniques. If need be, return to the station during breaks or after the formal teaching has ended and request additional instruction and practice. Although difficult to learn, the skills acquired will help you run more successful codes during your career.

REFERENCES

1. Guildner CW. Resuscitation-opening the airway: A comparative study of techniques for opening an airway obstructed by the tongue. *JACEP* 1976;5:588–590.
2. Morikawa S, Safar P, DeCarlo J. Influence of the head-jaw position on upper airway patency. *Anesthesiology* 1961;22:265–270.
3. Guidelines for cardiopulmonary resuscitation and emergency cardiac care. *JAMA* 1992;268:2171–2302.
4. Safar P. Cardiopulmonary cerebral resuscitation. Philadelphia: Saunders; Stavanger, Norway: Asmund S. Laerdal, 1981, p. 31.

5. Standards and guidelines for cardiopulmonary resuscitation and emergency cardiac care. *JAMA* 1980;155:2933.
6. Safar P. Cardiopulmonary cerebral resuscitation. Philadelphia: Saunders; Stavanger, Norway: Asmund S. Laerdal, 1981, p. 62.
7. Caroline NL. Emergency care in the streets. Third edition. Boston: Little, Brown, 1987, p. 223.
8. Jesudian MC, Harrison RR, Keenen RL, et al. Bag-valve-mask ventilation: Two rescuers are better than one. Preliminary report. *Crit Care Med* 1985;13: 122–123.

7 Essential Dysrhythmia Recognition

1. State the correct approach to basic interpretation of ECG rhythms and what constitutes a "normal" ECG.
2. Describe the normal duration of the QRS complex and the PR interval.
3. Identify the description of the following dysrhythmias:

   - Atrial tachycardia
   - Atrial flutter
   - Atrial fibrillation
   - Junctional rhythms
   - Ventricular escape rhythms
   - Accelerated ventricular rhythms
   - Torsades de pointes
   - Ventricular fibrillation
   - Asystole
   - First-degree AV heart block
   - Second-degree AV heart block
   - Third-degree heart block

Overview

Arrhythmia means the *absence* of rhythm. *Dysrhythmia* means the presence of an abnormal rhythm. Most people use these terms interchangeably, however.

One of the skills you will find necessary to have prior to taking an ACLS course is that of basic cardiac monitoring and rhythm interpretation. The pace and time frame of the program does not allow adequate time for the novice to become proficient enough with rhythm interpretation to complete the program without extreme difficulty. This chapter will review the basic steps for rhythm identification, describe some of the more common mistakes, and give a few helpful hints to use during rhythm identification.

Remember that an ECG will only tell you about the heart's electrical system. It cannot tell you about the patient's overall status. One key phrase that will be very helpful during the course of ACLS or whenever you are dealing with a patient is **Treat the patient, not the monitor!** The reality of the situation is that sometimes the patient is forgotten and health-care providers get hung up on the cardiac monitor screen. This should not happen.

Leads

Another common mistake is limiting yourself to only one lead for monitoring. A quote sometimes heard (or even spoken yourself) is, "I can't read that, it's not a Lead II." By using more than one lead, you can see the heart in a multidimensional view. You may not see P-waves in a Lead II, but they may be quite prominent in an MCL_1. Most monitoring devices used today have the capability to give you multiple leads, or views, by simply changing a switch on the machine. The four most common lead placements used for cardiac monitoring are Lead I, Lead II, Lead III, and MCL_1 (see Figures 7.1 and 7.2). Become familiar with their placement and with their normal looks and rules. The importance of using multiple leads to aid in accurate rhythm identification must be stressed.

Lead I   Positive electrode placed just
          below the left clavicle

          Negative electrode placed
          just below the right clavicle

          Provides information about
          the left lateral wall of the
          heart

Lead II   Positive electrode just below
          the left pectoral muscle

          Negative electrode just below
          the right clavicle

          Provides information about
          the inferior wall of the heart

Lead III Positive electrode placed just
          below the left pectoral
          muscle

          Negative electrode placed
          just below the left clavicle

          Provides information about
          the inferior wall of the heart

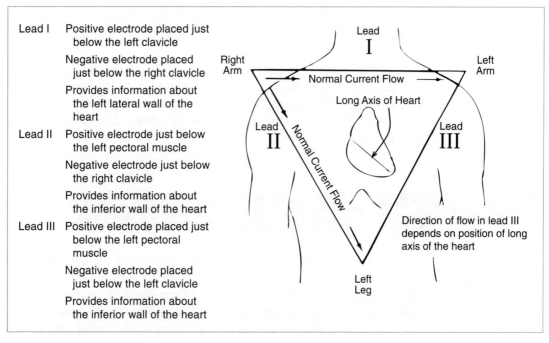

■ **Figure 7.1**   Location of chest Leads I, II, and III.

MCL   Negative electrode placed
       just below the left clavicle

       Positive electrode placed to
       the right of the sternum at
       the fourth intercostal space

       Provides information about
       the anterior wall of the heart

       May prove useful in assess-
       ing the width of the QRS
       complex to differentiate
       supraventricular tachycardia
       (SVT) from ventricular
       tachycardia (VT)

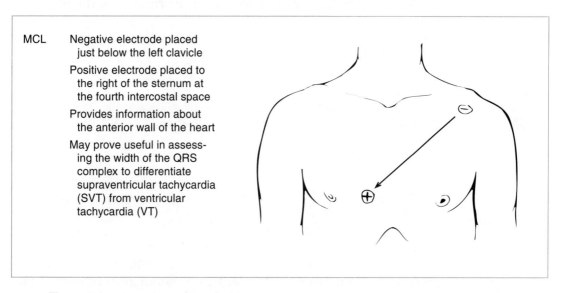

■ **Figure 7.2**   Location of Lead MCL.

Quick Look Paddles

Using the quick look capability of the defibrillator's paddles is generally recommended to initially rule out ventricular fibrillation or asystole. Continuous cardiac monitoring with the paddles, however, will be of a poor diagnostic quality due to artifact and poor patient-machine contact.

Looking

When you look at any rhythm strip, you should use the same format for identification, be it a simple rhythm or a more complex one. This will help you not to let some FLB (funny-looking beat) draw your attention away from the main problem. At times, health-care workers get into trouble with rhythm identification by doing something called a *shotgun approach* identification. This is where they see only one thing (such as a PVC) and then stop the rhythm analysis.

A recommended format is to look at the rhythm in the following fashion:

1. Regularity
2. Rate
3. P waves
4. PR interval (PRI)
5. QRS complexes
6. Ectopic beats

Regularity

This should be the starting ground for all rhythms, simple or complex. Without knowing the regularity, we cannot even get a good rate count. A regular rhythm will have equal spacing between each complex (S to S, QRS to QRS, etc.) regardless of the rate. This is an indication of the heart having only one pacer site (rule out all rhythms with multiple pacer sites). Irregular rhythms should be subdivided into regularly irregular or irregularly irregular.

Regularly Irregular Rhythms

These rhythms will have a pattern look to them. You could take three beats and lay them on top of the next three beats and they would have identical measurements (e.g., a sinus rhythm with trigeminal PVCs). Some other rhythms that have a regularly irregular look to them would be second-degree AV blocks, Type I (Wenckebach phenomenon); certain second-degree AV blocks, Type II; certain atrial flutters and pattern PACs, PJCs, PVCs with a regular underlying rhythm and sinus arrest/block.

Irregularly Irregular Rhythms

With these rhythms there will generally be multiple pacer sites (more than two) causing the irregular pattern. No matter how you cut them up you cannot find a group pattern with consistent measurements. Rhythms that fall into this group would be atrial fibrillation; ventricular fibrillation; wandering atrial pacemaker; certain atrial flutters; and nonpattern PACs, PJCs, PVCs.

Rate

The easiest way to deal with rate is to place the rate into one of three categories: slow, fast, or normal. A slow rate would be those rhythms with a ventricular rate below 60 beats per minute (rule out all the rhythms with the word *tachycardia* in them). A fast rate would include those rhythms with a ventricular rate greater than 100 beats per minute (rule out all those rhythms with the word *bradycardia* in them). If the rhythm has a ventricular rate somewhere between 60 to 100 beats per minute it would be within the normal range.

If you have a regularly occurring rhythm, you can count the rate by the number of large or small boxes between two QRS complexes. Remember that there are 300 large boxes (300 heavy lines/min), equivalent to 0.20 s each. There are also 1,500 smaller boxes in a 1-min strip with each small box on an ECG equal to 0.04s. The markers found at the top margin of the ECG paper are 3 s apart. You can estimate the rate by multiplying by 10 the number of QRS complexes within three markers (equal to a total of 6 s). An alternate way is to divide 300 by the number of heavy lines between complexes. For example, three heavy lines between complexes would equal a rate of 100, and four heavy lines a rate of 75.

P Wave

The P wave is the graphic display of atrial depolarization. There should be only one P wave for each QRS complex and each P wave should look like all the others. Different looking P waves usually means that the P wave is coming from a different pacer site. Rhythms that should come to mind with different looking P waves would include PACs, PJCs, and wandering atrial pacemaker. An MCL_1 lead will sometimes give you a better looking P wave than a Lead II. Having more P waves than QRS complexes is generally a sign of an AV block (discussed later in this chapter).

PR Interval

The PRI should be constant and within normal limits of 0.12 s to 0.20 s in times. A constant, prolonged PRI is usually a sign of a hold in the AV junction, such as seen with a first-degree AV block. A shorter

PRI (<0.20 s) can be a sign of a junctional beat (especially if the P wave is inverted). Inconsistent PRIs, with consistent looking P waves usually means an increasing hold in the AV junction as in a second degree AV block, Mobitz Type I, or a nonrelated AV relationship as in a third-degree AV block. Inconsistent PRIs associated with different looking P waves usually means PACs, PJCs, wandering atrial pacemakers, or atrial fibrillation.

QRS Complexes

The QRS complexes are the graphic representation of ventricular depolarization. A normal QRS will have a measurement of <0.12 s. A wider than normal QRS complex can mean it is ventricular in nature or aberrantly conducted. If each QRS complex is associated with a P wave, it is generally considered to be sinus in nature (regardless of the width). A rhythm with a wide QRS complex and no associated P wave should be considered ventricular until proven otherwise.

Ectopic Beats

Confusion occurs when ectopic beats occur. Ectopic beats should be overlooked for the most part until the underlying rhythm can be determined. After identifying the underlying rhythm, the next stop will be to identify the origin of the ectopic beat. Each ectopic beat should be classified as atrial, junctional, ventricular, or aberrant in origin. If the ectopic beat has a P wave associated with it, a normal or longer-than-normal PRI, and a normal QRS complex, it will probably be atrial in nature (PAC). If the ectopic beat has a P wave, a shorter-than-normal PRI, and a normal QRS complex, it is probably junctional (PJC) especially in the presence of an inverted P wave. Some PJCs will not have a P wave associated with them (consequently, no PRI). An ectopic beat that does not have a P wave associated with it, no PRI, and a wider-than-normal QRS complex is generally ventricular (PVC). A wide QRS complex with a normal P wave and normal PRI is generally an aberrantly (outside of normal) conducted complex.

Identifying the Rhythm

As stated before, we take all the information gathered from the ECG or monitor and eliminate those rhythms that do not fit the information. Generally, the first part of the rhythm's name will identify the pacer site while the second would identify the rate. If we were to identify a rhythm as a sinus bradycardia, we could determine that the pacer site was in the sinus node and the rate was less than 60 beats per minute. Ventricular fibrillation would identify the pacer site as being in the ventricles, while the rate would be greater than 300 beats per minute.

Sinus Rhythm

The key finding to any sinus rhythm will be an associated P wave with each QRS complex. Each P wave will look the same and the PRI will be within a normal limit. The QRS complex can be outside the normal limit (usually a sign of an intraventricular conduction delay), but as long as the P wave is associated it has to be sinus in nature. Figure 7.3 shows an ECG tracing of sinus rhythm.

If the rate is below 60 beats per minute, it would be considered a *sinus bradycardia*. If the rate is between 60 and 100 beats per minute, a *sinus rhythm*. After the rate reaches greater than 100 beats per minute, it would be a *sinus tachycardia*. Most sinus tachycardias will have a rate between 100 and 160 beats per minute.

There can be a slight change in the regularity pattern, usually associated with the patient's respiration. This would be a sign of a *sinus arrhythmia,* generally not a life-threatening rhythm by itself (see Figure 7.4).

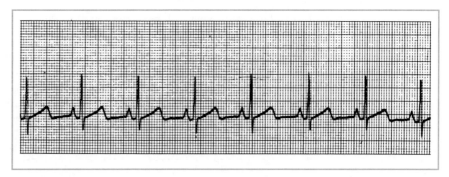

■ **Figure 7.3**   Sinus rhythm.

Sinus Arrhythmia

Sinus arrhythmias usually have a rate of 60 to 100 beats per minute. The rate can vary but is generally *irregular*. P waves are upright and uniform in appearance with one P wave preceding *each* QRS complex. The PRI is usually 0.12 s to 0.20 s but can vary between beats causing an irregular pulse (see Figure 7.4).

Atrial Tachycardia

With atrial tachycardia, the P wave usually will not be seen because of the fast rate (increased heart rate means less recovery time, shorter R-R cycles). The identity is primarily based on the rhythm being regu-

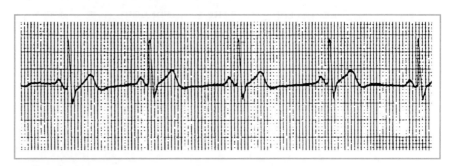

■ **Figure 7.4**   Sinus arrhythmia.

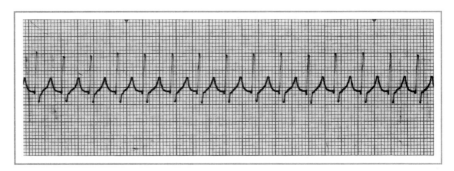

■ **Figure 7.5**   Atrial tachycardia.

lar, the rate between 150 and 250 beats per minute, and the QRS complex being within normal limits. Occasionally, a narrow complex ventricular tachycardia with a rate greater than 150 may be confused with an atrial tachycardia, especially if using only one lead.

Some people will generally call any atrial tachycardia paroxysmal atrial tachycardia (PAT). In order to have a true PAT you will need to see the beginning of the tachycardia, as paroxysmal means sudden onset (see Figure 7.5).

Atrial Flutter

In atrial flutter there is only one pacer site outside of the sinus node. This pacer site will generally have a discharge rate of between 220 and 350 times per minute. This fast rate and being outside of the sinus node will cause the P wave (flutter wave) to take on the "sawtooth" or "picket fence" look.

The atrial rate will be consistent while the ventricular response may be either consistent or inconsistent. This depends on how many atrial discharges can "get through" to cause a ventricular response. The QRS complexes with atrial flutter will generally be consistent in appearance regardless of the width (see Figure 7.6).

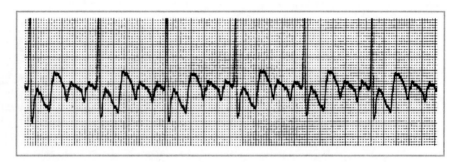

■ **Figure 7.6   Atrial flutter.**

Atrial Fibrillation

With atrial fibrillation, there will be multiple pacer sites outside of the sinus node discharging in an irregular pattern. The atrial discharge rate will be greater than 300 times per minute and because of the different pacer sites the fibrillatory waves will also look different when seen.

Because of the multiple pacer sites and the rapid irregular atrial rate, the ventricular response is generally irregular. Thus, the famous irregularly irregular rhythm. Atrial fibrillation can be subcategorized into controlled and uncontrolled atrial fibrillation. If the ventricular response is 100 or less, it is usually considered to be controlled. If the ventricular rate is greater than 100 discharges per minute, it is defined as being uncontrolled atrial fibrillation (see Figure 7.7).

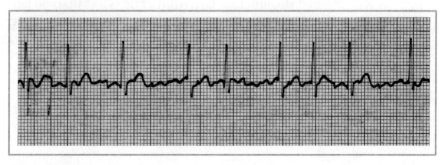

■ **Figure 7.7   Atrial fibrillation.**

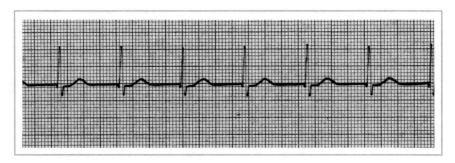

■ **Figure 7.8**   Junctional rhythm (accelerated).

Junctional Rhythm

Key findings of most junctional rhythms will be the absence of an associated P wave to the normal-looking QRS complex. P waves may be visible with certain types of junctional rhythms. Some junctional rhythms can have P waves in front of the QRS complex, but the PRI will be shorter than normal (<0.12 s) and the P wave may be inverted due to retrograde depolarization. Other junctional rhythms may have P waves following the QRS complexes (within the ST segment). Again, these P waves may also be inverted.

The QRS complexes will generally be within the normal limits (<0.12 s) due to the depolarization process being initiated from above the ventricles. Wide complexed junctional rhythms will need an in-depth study to rule out a ventricular rhythm.

If the junctional rhythm's rate is less than 60 beats per minute, it is generally classified as a *junctional escape rhythm*. If the rate is between 60 and 100 beats per minute, it will be classified as an *accelerated junctional rhythm*. If the rate is greater than 100, it is classified as a junctional tachycardia (see Figure 7.8).

Ventricular Rhythm

By far, ventricular rhythms are the most common cause of sudden cardiac death. One of the easiest ways to identify a ventricular rhythm will be by the wide QRS complexes. Because the primary pacer site is outside of the normal conduction pathway and located within the ventricles, it will take a longer time period for the impulse to complete its travel. This time delay will be reflected by the increased width of the QRS complex (ventricular depolarization).

In addition to the abnormal QRS complexes, ventricular rhythms will not have an associated P wave (atrial depolarization) with each cardiac cycle. The dissociation between the atriums and ventricular areas may be due to either an escape rhythm or by an irritable area(s).

Ventricular Escape Rhythm (Idio-ventricular)

Characteristics of a ventricular escape rhythm would include absence of P waves or nonassociated P waves, wide QRS complexes, and a regular pattern (irregular pattern may be present with a slow rate) due to only one pacer site. If the rate is between 20 and 40 beats per minute, it is classified as a ventricular escape rhythm.

Accelerated Ventricular Rhythm

If the rate is between 40 and 100 beats per minute with the same characteristics as above, it is classified as an accelerated ventricular escape rhythm.

Ventricular Tachycardia

If the ventricular rate exceeds 100 beats per minute and has the other characteristics of a ventricular rhythm, it will be identified as a ventricular tachycardia (rate will generally be >150) (see Figure 7.9).

Torsades de Pointes

This is a special type of ventricular tachycardia that is characterized by a changing of the amplitude and direction of the electrical forces. This type of ventricular tachycardia will need to be treated differently

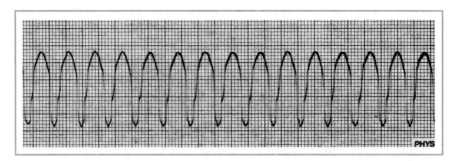

■ **Figure 7.9**   Ventricular tachycardia.

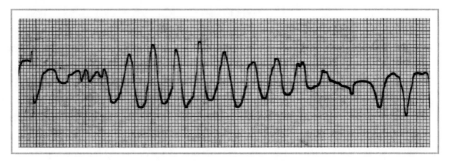

■ **Figure 7.10**   Torsades de pointes.

than classical VT (see Figure 7.10). This dysrhythmia can be caused by medications (e.g., tricyclic antidepressants, phenothiazines), electrolyte abnormalities, liquid protein diets, mitral valve prolapse, marked bradycardia, ischemia, or myocarditis.

Ventricular Fibrillation

When there are multiple pacer sites within the ventricles (usually due to irritation), no common pattern can be seen. This will result in ventricular fibrillation. Ventricular fibrillation is identified by the lack of coordinated ventricular depolarization (QRS complexes) and no atrial activity (P waves). Artifact such as that caused by a loose elec-

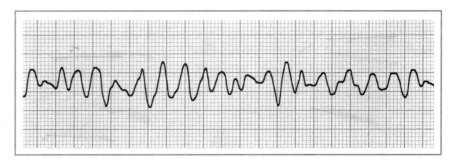

■ **Figure 7.11**   **Ventricular fibrillation.**

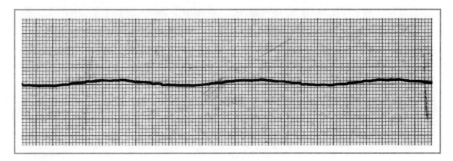

■ **Figure 7.12**   Asystole.

trode can mimic ventricular fibrillation and should be ruled out immediately by assessing the patient (see Figure 7.11).

Asystole

The one rhythm all health-care providers should be able to readily identify is asystole. This rhythm is identified by the lack of any electrical activity (flat line). Always confirm asystole by changing to a second lead since occasionally it is difficult to delineate between a fine ventricular fibrillation and asystole.

In the presence of an occasional escape beat (rate usually <10) it may be called an *agonal rhythm* or a *dying heart*. Both rhythms would be classified as asystole (see Figure 7.12), although many people do not, by definition, treat a rhythm classified as agonal.

AV Heart Blocks

Probably the hardest type of rhythm to identify is what type of heart block you are dealing with. We'll show you a couple of simple items to help you identify the type of block with a high success rate.

First-Degree AV Block

A first-degree AV block does not actually "block" any electrical activity, but it delays the electrical impulse through the AV node. This rhythm has an underlying sinus rhythm with a prolonged but constant PRI (>0.20 s). The PRI is prolonged due to an increased hold in the AV junction, but still with a one-to-one relationship (one P wave to each QRS complex). If the patient is symptomatic, it will generally be due to the rate being abnormal (bradycardia or tachycardia) (see Figure 7.13).

Other Heart Blocks

The one common finding in any of the other AV blocks will be the presence of more P waves than QRS complexes. One place to remember to look for P waves is in the T wave. The most common reason for misshapen T waves is the presence of atrial activity hidden within.

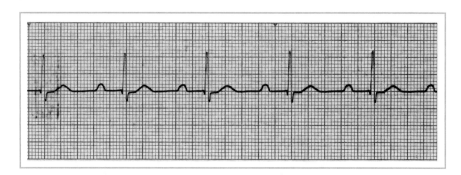

■ **Figure 7.13**   First-degree AV block.

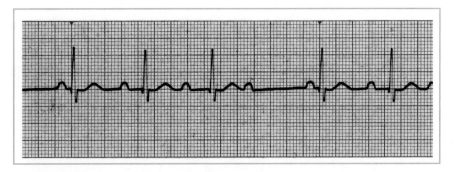

Figure 7.14 Second-degree AV block: Mobitz type I.

Second-Degree AV Blocks

Mobitz Type I (Wenckebach)

With a second-degree AV block, Type I, you will find an increasing PRI with the conducted P wave. This increase is due to an increased hold within the AV junction, delaying the depolarization process. This hold increases to the point that a ventricular response (QRS complex) is dropped. This causes an irregular rhythm that may be regularly irregular or irregularly irregular. This can be further classified by stating the conduction ratio of atrial response to ventricular response (e.g., 4:3, four P waves to three QRS complexes) (see Figure 7.14).

Mobitz Type II (classical)

This type of block occurs when certain atrial depolarizations cannot be conducted through the AV junction to cause ventricular depolarization. The P waves that do get through to conduct (in front of the QRS complexes) will have a consistent PRI. This rhythm will again be irregular due to the nonconducted P waves and may be regularly irregular or irregularly irregular. In other words, the PRI is prolonged but constant with occasional dropped beats (see Figure 7.15).

Third-Degree AV Block

Third-degree AV blocks are identified again by the presence of more P waves than QRS complexes. This will be coupled with no correlation between the atrial activity (P waves) and the ventricular activity (QRS

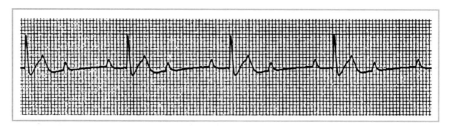

■ **Figure 7.15**   Second-degree AV block: Mobitz type II.

complexes). In other words, the PRI will be inconsistent while the R to R will be consistent. The P to P will be consistent because the sinus node will be discharging normally, but the impulses will not be conducted through the AV junction to cause ventricular depolarization (inconsistent PRI). The R to R will be consistent because the ventricular depolarization will be controlled by a secondary pacer site below the atrial and AV area.

Third-degree AV blocks can be further identified by the location of the secondary pacer site. If the QRS complexes are within normal limits, the pacer site will be located above the ventricles, usually in the junction. If the QRS complexes are greater than normal, the pacer site will be located within the ventricles (see Figure 7.16). An AV Block Identification chart can be found in Figure 7.17.

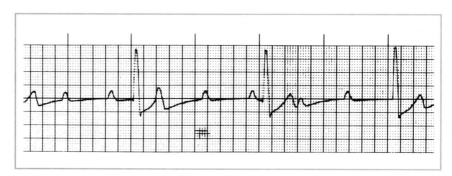

■ **Figure 7.16**   Third-degree AV block.

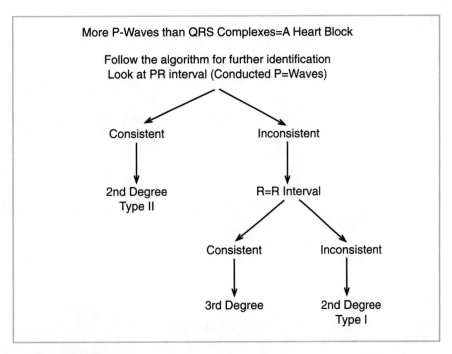

More P-Waves than QRS Complexes=A Heart Block

Follow the algorithm for further identification
Look at PR interval (Conducted P=Waves)

Consistent   Inconsistent

2nd Degree   R=R Interval
Type II

Consistent   Inconsistent

3rd Degree   2nd Degree
Type I

■ **Figure 7.17**   **AV block identification.**

Summary

Rhythm recognition is an integral part of the ACLS course. You *must* be familiar with the basic required rhythms *before* you come to the first day of class. Dysrhythmia recognition is the very essence of emergency cardiac care. Unless you are able to diagnose the dysrhythmia, you cannot proceed with the appropriate intervention. If you know you will have difficulty with this section, make sure you review the required dysrhythmias at least one month prior to the course.

Notes

What's Important about Myocardial Infarction

Objectives

1. Discuss the pathophysiological events that can lead to an MI.
2. Describe the physiology of flow regulation for the coronary system and etiologies for alterations in the normal supply to the myocardium.
3. List three clinical manifestations of CAD.
4. Describe the usual treatment of acute MIs.

Overview

In the United States there has been a dramatic reduction in heart disease mortality in the past 20 years. About seven million people in the United States currently have CAD. However, in men and women heart disease remains the leading cause of death, even though there is a reduction in the major risk factors of high blood pressure, obesity, elevated cholesterol, and smoking. Many times, the mortality from cardiovascular disease can be lowered with a change in lifestyle and this modification can enhance the prevention and management of CAD. This chapter will provide a brief overview to the physiology of normal cardiac function and the pathophysiology associated with disease states.

Coronary Arteries and Veins

Adequate oxygen must be supplied to the cells of the myocardium in order to supply an energy substrate for continuous work and adequate cardiac output. Elevated temperatures, stress, and exercise cause increased workload on the heart initiating increased coronary blood flow that can be stimulated intrinsically or extrinsically through several mechanisms to provide vital oxygen to the mitochondria of the myocardium.

The blood is routed to the cells of the myocardium via the right and left coronary arteries and these arteries come off the aorta just above the aortic valve. Both arteries branch out densely throughout the musculature into very small capillary beds providing sufficient oxygen and nourishment to the myocardium.

In the event of a chronic obstruction (e.g., atherosclerotic plaque) to blood flow in a branch of the coronary artery system, collateral channels expand and allow renewed flow to the affected areas. The cardiac veins take blood and spent products of energy metabolism and return it to the right atrium to join blood returning from the vena cavas.

Flow Regulation

The perfusion pressure, vascular resistance, and coronary oxygen saturation (oxygen tension) provide the main determinants of flow in the coronary system. Coronary oxygen tension is believed to be the major determinant for coronary blood flow. Myocardial oxygen tension decreases as exercise increases and increased oxygen is needed to supply the myocardium. This, in turn, causes a fall in coronary vascular resistance, which increases coronary flow, which thus provides an increased myocardial oxygen tension for the cells. This is an autoregulated mechanism that adjusts coronary vascular resistance to accommodate an increased demand for myocardial oxygen tension during variations in physiological needs (e.g., due to increased exercise). Therefore, myocardial oxygen consumption is directly related to coronary blood flow. To provide this increase in myocardial oxygen for increased work, there is initially an increase in heart rate, which results in an increase in the cardiac output.

Alteration in Flow

Atheromatous accumulations in the walls of the arteries cause a decrease in total flow through the vessel. These lesions extend out through most of the vessel and can become calcified, thus providing only a minimal trickle of blood to the cells in the area served by this vessel. These arteries may occlude totally if the process continues. Spasm can also decrease blood flow through coronary arteries.

Regulation of Cardiac Output

Regulation of cardiac output occurs due to the following factors: (1) *preload*; (2) *afterload*; (3) *heart rate, rhythm, and stroke volume*; (4) *myocardial contractility*; and (5) *ejection fraction*. These major components of cardiac output work to maintain the flow at an optimal level. The energy developed during contraction of the myocardium is a function of the muscle length just prior to contraction. This muscle length is called *preload* and is needed to stretch the muscle from its precontraction length. Preload is obtained or generated by the return of venous blood. When that venous return is greater than normal, then the very next beat will increase to a higher stroke volume.

Afterload can be thought of as total peripheral resistance in the vascular system that the heart must work against in order to push the blood through the great vessels and into the tissues. The opposition to left ventricular ejection *into* the aorta is termed *afterload*.

Cardiac output is kept constant when the heart rate is well within its normal limits because the stroke volume remains the same as do the afterload and preload. Physiologic changes that impinge on the heart rate, stroke volume, or any of the other determinants can cause a decrease in cardiac output, which worsens the myocardial contractility and decreases cardiac ejection fraction.

End-diastolic volume represents the volume that remains in the heart at the end of systole. The *ejection fraction* is equal to the stroke volume divided by the left ventricular end-diastolic volume. This measure is a function of the heart as a pump and can be determined via several measures, both invasive and noninvasive.

Coronary Spasm

Coronary spasm can cause sudden and severe decreases in coronary blood flow to vital myocardial areas. Spasm most commonly presents as angina at rest with ST elevation, and transient ventricular ectopy, and conduction abnormalities may occur. A decrease in flow to the myocardial vascular system can also be caused by stenosis from an atherosclerotic plaque that is aggravated by a concurrent coronary artery spasm at the site of the atherosclerotic plaque. The vast majority of patients with spasm also have fixed coronary obstructions and may, therefore, also have a history of exertional angina. Up to 20% of these patients have an MI in the first six months following the development of clinical findings consistent with coronary spasm.

Stenosis

Generally, when the stenosis is minimal, usually less than 55%, no significant decrease in flow is initially apparent. However, over time, as the stenotic area becomes greater and the oxygen demand increases during exercise or stress, angina, MI, or sudden death can occur.

Occlusion

Total occlusion of the artery results in diminished or absent circulation, causing a decrease in oxygen to the mitochondria and inability of the tissue to trade off spent products of energy metabolism, (e.g., carbon dioxide, lactic acid).

The right coronary artery (RCA) supplies the anterior and posterior walls of the right ventricles, the right atrium, and the sino-atrial node. It also supplies the posterior one third of the inter-ventricular septum, the AV node, the upper half of the inter-atrial septum, and the posterior base of the left ventricle.

The left coronary artery (LCA) supplies the left anterior descending, diagonal, septal, marginal, and circumflex branches. The left anterior descending provides blood to the anterior septum and the circumflex provides the left ventricle and branches through the coronary sulcus all the way to the posterior descending branch of the RCA. These branches of the LCA provide needed blood to the entire left ventricle. It also supplies branches to the anterior two thirds of the inter-ventricular septum, the anterior left margin of the free wall of the right ventricle, the apex, the lower half of the inter-atrial septum, and the left atrium.

It is important to remember that coronary artery spasms, whether of the right or left, can produce intermittent chest pain even at rest and the patient may develop a sense of impending doom. The administration of nitroglycerin (NTG) and the relief of the spasm and pain, may be a confirmation of the presence of spasm in these patients.

Risk Factors for Predisposition for CAD

The following risk factors cannot be changed:
- Male
- Age
- Family history of CAD

The following risk factors can be controlled or modified:
- Hypertension
- Hypercholesterolemia
- Diabetes mellitus
- Obesity
- Sedentary lifestyle
- Type A behavior and stress
- Smoking

Multiple risk factors increase the morbidity and mortality progressively. Other potential risk factors include contraceptive use and being a postmenopausal female. Risk factor modification is the paramount goal in the prevention of CAD, whether or not subsequent treatment is medical or surgical. Lifestyle change is the key to limiting the cumulative effects of CAD.

Clinical Manifestations of CAD

The clinical manifestations of CAD include cardiac arrhythmias, angina, acute MI, heart failure, and sudden death (usually due to an arrhythmia). The clinician's clinical acumen, which includes an understanding of early management of acute MI and its life-threatening complications, can help reduce the long-term mortality and morbidity that accompanies an acute MI.

Cardiac Arrhythmias

It is important for the clinician and all ACLS providers to be able to immediately recognize cardiac arrhythmias, especially those potentially lethal arrhythmias, and respond with the appropriate intervention. Anti-arrhythmic agents must be initiated immediately and used accurately in this setting if the clinician hopes to influence and stabilize an acutely ischemic myocardium. Arrhythmogenic mechanisms can also be initiated by a change in the electrolytes as well as mineral composition of the blood. Cardiac arrhythmias seen postinfarct are a potentially lethal complication.

Angina

Myocardial ischemia, which results in decreased oxygen supply, produces angina. This chest pain or discomfort can be substernal or diffuse across the chest. Some patients describe it as a vice or heaviness to their chest, which begins to intensify very rapidly. The pain, as described, is said to radiate into either arm or shoulder, to the neck, jaw, or back. Other patients note they have a feeling of indigestion or bloating in the epigastric or abdominal area.

The AHA recommends that a patient with known angina pectoris seek emergency medical care if chest pain is not relieved by three NTG tablets over a 10-minute period. In a person with previously unrecognized coronary disease, the persistence of suspicious chest pain for two minutes or longer is an indication for emergency medical assistance, as recommended by the AHA. In many patients, the initial chest pain may be denied or not mentioned to family members or co-workers. As a result, hours may pass before the patient seeks needed medical attention. Clinicians realize that it is the prompt response to a cardiopulmonary event that will lessen the effect of MI and decrease the mortality and morbidity associated with sudden death.

Physical exercise and stress can trigger angina, but anginal pain can also occur at rest, depending on the severity of the CAD. During exercise, myocardial oxygen demand increases and severe CAD limits the ability of the coronary arteries to provide an increased oxygen supply and angina then results. Unstable angina generally develops in individuals who have severely stenosed coronary arteries and they are at high risk for an MI. Usually during unstable angina, there is an acceleration of heart rate to provide more blood because of the increase in myocardial oxygen consumption. There is generally a marked ST depression that usually can be reversed after NTG is administered.

Sudden Death

Sudden cardiac death can occur in patients who may have had no precipitating cardiac symptoms. *Sudden cardiac death* as defined by the World Health Organization is death that occurs within 24 hours after onset of precipitating symptoms and may be due to a sudden arrhythmic death or myocardial failure/infarction. Most of these cardiac-related deaths are due to valvular heart disease, ischemic and coronary disease, congestive cardiomyopathies, or hypertensive heart disease. These conditions can cause sudden arrhythmic death with the development of fatal ventricular fibrillation.

Myocardial Infarction

Myocardial ischemia can lead to necrosis or death of heart muscle and is called *myocardial infarction*. This necrosis is the result of a severe narrowing of the coronary arteries due to atherosclerotic plaques with or without accompanying thrombus formation and/or spasm.

Clinicians are keenly aware that prior to the infarction, arrhythmogenic events are in progress and can happen acutely and must be recognized immediately or they could become life-threatening. Occlusions of the coronary artery that occur closer to the main lumen obviously cause greater damage than if the occlusion were in a more distal smaller branch. As mentioned earlier, collateral blood supply is very important because it can help carry blood around these occluded areas.

The treatment of MIs includes placement of the patient in an intensive care unit setting, ECG monitoring, pain relief, sedation if indicated, thrombolytic therapy if appropriate, anticoagulation for dissemination of the thrombosis, and complication management. In reviewing thrombolytic therapy, which should begin immediately and preferrably within the first hour following an acute MI, it provides appropriate treatment for the management of thrombosis, which results in coronary occlusion. This action may prevent further necrosis and life-threatening complications associated with an MI, including cardiac arrhythmias, heart failure, pericarditis, myocardial rupture, thromboembolism, and ventricular aneurysm. Factors that potentially worsen life-threatening complications of MI include history of a previous MI, complex ventricular arrhythmias that occur after an MI, systolic hypotension, heart failure, older age, and the presence of a left bundle branch block. American Heart Association recommendations for treatment of acute MIs are in Figure 8.1.

Heart Failure

A decrease in myocardial contractility results in congestive heart failure (CHF). The heart failure is indicated by orthopnea, persistent cough, difficulty breathing, an enlarged liver, cyanosis, and edema, as well as peripheral congestion. During the physical examination of a patient in CHF, you may detect weak heart tones, systolic or diastolic murmurs, a pericardial friction rub, ventricular enlargement, and cardiac arrhythmias. In essence, heart failure is the inability to provide adequate perfusion due to decreased cardiac output to the tissues of the body. Decreasing cardiac output also increases the likelihood that lactic acidosis will develop in the tissues.

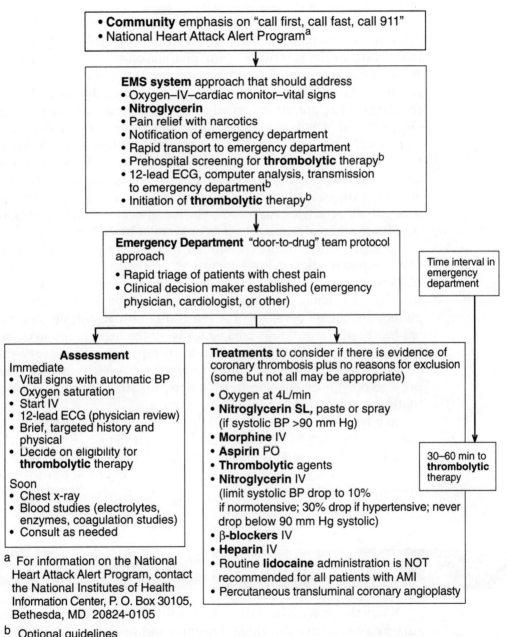

• **Community** emphasis on "call first, call fast, call 911"
• National Heart Attack Alert Program[a]

↓

EMS system approach that should address
• Oxygen–IV–cardiac monitor–vital signs
• **Nitroglycerin**
• Pain relief with narcotics
• Notification of emergency department
• Rapid transport to emergency department
• Prehospital screening for **thrombolytic** therapy[b]
• 12-lead ECG, computer analysis, transmission
  to emergency department[b]
• Initiation of **thrombolytic** therapy[b]

↓

Emergency Department "door-to-drug" team protocol
approach
• Rapid triage of patients with chest pain
• Clinical decision maker established (emergency
  physician, cardiologist, or other)

Time interval in
emergency
department

Assessment
Immediate
• Vital signs with automatic BP
• Oxygen saturation
• Start IV
• 12-lead ECG (physician review)
• Brief, targeted history and
  physical
• Decide on eligibility for
  thrombolytic therapy

Soon
• Chest x-ray
• Blood studies (electrolytes,
  enzymes, coagulation studies)
• Consult as needed

Treatments to consider if there is evidence of
coronary thrombosis plus no reasons for exclusion
(some but not all may be appropriate)

• Oxygen at 4L/min
• **Nitroglycerin SL,** paste or spray
  (if systolic BP >90 mm Hg)
• **Morphine** IV
• **Aspirin** PO
• **Thrombolytic** agents
• **Nitroglycerin** IV
  (limit systolic BP drop to 10%
  if normotensive; 30% drop if hypertensive; never
  drop below 90 mm Hg systolic)
• **β-blockers** IV
• **Heparin** IV
• Routine **lidocaine** administration is NOT
  recommended for all patients with AMI
• Percutaneous transluminal coronary angioplasty

30–60 min to
thrombolytic
therapy

[a] For information on the National
Heart Attack Alert Program, contact
the National Institutes of Health
Information Center, P. O. Box 30105,
Bethesda, MD 20824-0105

[b] Optional guidelines

■ **Figure 8.1**   Acute myocardial infarction (MI) algorithm. Recommendations for early
management of patients with chest pain and possible acute MI. Reproduced with permission. CPR Issue, JAMA, October 28, 1993. © American
Heart Association.

Following an MI, hemodynamic monitoring is essential to allow the clinician to determine whether the patient has any CHF and the degree. Depending on the severity, varying pharmacological agents are used. These agents attempt to improve hemodynamic measurements, which will limit the extent of the heart failure. Generally, during periods of rest, the cardiac output is normal in the early stages of heart failure. Over a period of time, the heart failure may worsen and be associated with a decreased cardiac output. The patient may need to be evaluated with a chest x-ray to denote pulmonary venous dilation, cardiac silhouette enlargement, and congested lung fields. The patient may also have an echocardiogram to measure heart chamber size and the contractile state of both ventricles. An echo can be useful in evaluating patients for the presence of pericardial effusions or valvular heart disease.

Cardiac catheterization is another method of evaluation. A right heart catheterization using a Swan-Ganz catheter can provide clinicians with the pulmonary artery wedge pressure that indirectly measures left ventricular and diastolic pressure and the cardiac output. As pulmonary edema develops or worsens, the cardiac output falls. The left heart catheterization is used basically for the determination of any surgically correctable lesions, ventricular septal defects, aneurysms, and, most importantly, the coronary anatomy. A left ventriculogram can also provide an ejection fraction determination, which can quantitatively predict the amount of heart failure.

In a transmural acute MI, the ECG can present with pathologic Q waves, which may not become apparent until the day following the infarction. There are also non-Q wave infarctions, which may have pronounced ST segment depression or T wave inversion but without the presence of Q waves.

Serum Cardiac Enzyme Changes

When the cells of the myocardium become injured, they release an enzyme system into the blood. Enzymes and isoenzymes can be isolated and measured. Creatine phosphokinase (CPK) and CPK-MB isoenzymes are evaluated. The CPK generally peaks within the first 24 hours and returns to normal within three to four days. It may also be elevated in other conditions, especially those associated with tissue injury. CPK isoenzymes can help to rule out noncardiac causes of these elevations. CPK-MB is designed to detect myocardial necrosis more specifically than the CPK alone. It usually peaks within 18 to 24 hours and generally returns to normal within two to four days. CPK-MB comprises a larger portion of the myocardium and is rarely seen in skeletal muscle. There may also be increases in the SGOT, LDH, and LDH isoenzyme levels that can assist in diagnosing an acute MI. The LDH isoenzyme has a greater specificity for the myocardial tissue as does the CPK-MB isoenzyme. The others have less specificity because they may increase in other conditions of muscle injury.

Pericarditis

Pericarditis may complicate a patient recovering from an acute MI and signs and symptoms include chest pain/discomfort, fever, and a pericardial rub. The pain/discomfort is usually in the center of the chest, may be referred to the back, and is often pleuritic in nature (i.e., aggravated by inspiration or coughing). The pain/discomfort is generally relieved, at least partially, by sitting up and leaning forward. Tachycardia is also generally associated with pericarditis as well as ST elevation and a low-voltage QRS if there is an effusion.

Summary

Myocardial infarction can be treated effectively in many patients. Survival may be followed by a return to normal activities within eight weeks, although any elective surgery and flying should be delayed for at least six months. Cardiac rehabilitation programs are an important aspect of the post-MI patient's management and should be strongly encouraged with active participation of both spouse and family. Modification of risk factors, exercise, and medical follow-up should be emphasized in order to maximize the chance for the patient who has suffered an acute MI to return to a fairly normal lifestyle.

During the ACLS course, it is important to remember that MIs can lead to disturbances in the ability of the body to pump blood (e.g., hypo-tension), may affect heart rate, and can lead to potentially fatal arrhythmias (e.g., VT, VF, asystole). As such, the pathophysiology is important to understand in terms of the complex resuscitation and postresuscitation problems one might encounter during mega code/case-based teaching scenarios presented to you.

Bibliography

Overview

Yusuf S, Wittes J, Friedman L. Overview of results of randomized clinical trials in heart disease, I: Treatments following myocardial infarction. *JAMA* 1988;260:2088–2093.

O'Rourke GW, Greene NM. Autonomic blockade and the resting heart rate in man. *Am Heart J* 1970;80:469–474.

Reich-Atkins S. Matters of the heart: Coronary artery disease in women. *J Am Acad Phys Assts* 1992;5:241–248.

Coronary Perfusion

Rushmer RF. *Cardiovascular dynamics,* fourth edition. Philadelphia: Saunders, 1976; pp.36–75, 351–366.

Timmis AD. *Cardiology.* New York: Gower Medical, 1985, pp. 16–34.

ACLS Textbook, third edition. Dallas: American Heart Association, 1994.

Cardiac Output

Little RC. *Physiology of the heart and circulation,* third edition. Chicago: Year Book Medical, 1985, pp. 152–181.

Prophylactic Treatment

Dunn HM, McComb JM, Kinney CD, et al. Prophylactic lidocaine in the early phase of suspected myocardial infarction. *Am Heart J* 1985;110:353–362.

MacMahon S, Collins R, Peto R, et al. Effects of prophylactic lidocaine in suspected acute myocardial infarction: An overview of results from the randomized controlled trials. *JAMA* 1988;260:1910–1916.

Olson DW, Thompson BM, Darin JC, et al. A randomized comparison study of bretylium tosylate and lidocaine in resuscitation of patients from out-of-hospital ventricular fibrillation in a paramedic system. *Ann Emerg Med* 1984;13(pt 2):807–810.

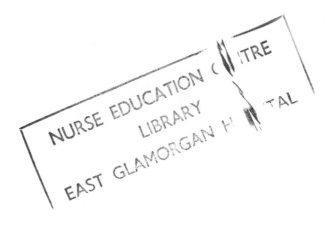

Notes

9 Electrical Therapy and How to Use It

9

Objectives

1. Describe the use of defibrillation versus synchronized cardioversion.
2. State the correct energy levels for use in defibrillation and cardioversion.
3. List the indications for pacing.
4. Identify the uses and limitations of automated external defibrillators.

Overview

Rapid defibrillation remains the major determinant of survival in cardiac arrest due to VF. It is critical that the health care provider fully understand and be comfortable with the proper use of defibrillation and cardioversion.

After completing an ACLS course, it is important to remember that each hospital, clinic, emergency department, or ambulance may have *different* models of defibrillators. Even though all models basically function similarly, each one has its own particular variations on design, button locations, and other features. It is *critical* for you to be familiar with the unit you will be expected to use during a code! Take a few minutes each time you are assigned to a code team, ambulance, or ACLS course mega code/case-based teaching station to review the particular features of the machine so you will not have to try and do it during an emergency or in the ACLS testing situation.

Unsynchronized Defibrillation

The chief indication for use of defibrillation is VF and pulseless VT. Defibrillation is *not* the treatment of choice for true asystole (remember, true asystole is not "very fine" VF!). The main theory of use is that defibrillation is to depolarize all individual cardiac cells, which then enables them to repolarize at the same time with subsequent return of coordinated cardiac contractility. An unsynchronized defibrillation will deliver energy in joules (= watt-seconds), where the energy (joules) = power (watts) × duration (seconds). Current (in amps) is what defibrillates the myocardium (not voltage) and the transthoracic resistance (TTR) to the passage of current can affect the amount of energy actually reaching the myocardial tissue. The TTR can be affected by the time between defibrillation attempts and the number of shocks delivered to the chest wall. A minimum of 30 to 40 amps across the myocardium is generally needed to obtain the desired effect.

The recommended energy levels for adults are as follows:

Initial attempt	200 joules
Second attempt	200 to 300 joules
Third attempt	360 joules
Subsequent attempts	360 joules

Note: Escalation of energy only occurs if the prior energy level was unsuccessful in terminating the ventricular rhythm. If recurring episodes of VF are successfully ended by a shock of 200 joules, the energy levels are *not* raised. If the rhythm returns and is broken by a low-level shock, then there is no need to raise the level of energy even if it is the 15th shock. Shocking a patient is not an innocuous activity. We consider each shock administered as potentially damaging to the conduction system. We try to keep energy levels as low as possible, while still remaining effective—a true cost-benefit relationship.

There is no clear-cut relationship between weight and energy level in adults, although weight can affect energy needed in infants and small children.

Operator Techniques

Paddle placement
- Right: Midclavicular line just below clavicle
- Left: Midaxillary line about the 6th rib (you may need to move the arm for correct placement)

Paddle pressure/contact
- 25 lbs (11 kg)
- Use firm pressure (avoid gaps/spaces under the paddle)
- Adjust paddle for best fit to the contour of patient's chest
- Avoid excessive jelly (can cause bridging if pressure/contact not correct)
- **Never** use alcohol pads! (danger of fire)

Defibrillator pads
- Clean and help prevent bridging of current
- Packaging can be hard to open in an emergency
- Can slide off patient's chest
- Can curl up under the paddle

Saline-soaked gauze pads
- Inexpensive
- Excess saline on the skin will also conduct the current during countershock and can cause burns to the skin
- Can also slide off patient's chest

Operator safety
- Avoid *all* patient contact
- After calling "all clear," make sure everyone has heard you and has moved away from the patient. Scan the *entire* area!
- Avoid allowing your fingers to touch the paddles
- Be sure that your stethoscope is not touching the patient

Patient safety
- Burns can result from poor technique (poor contact/pressure/jell)
- Avoid electrical arcing

Internal Defibrillation

- Internal paddles cup the heart in much the same position as external paddles so that the current will traverse the myocardial tissue
- Energy levels are much lower—5 joules (J) and then increase gradually to maximum of 40 to 50 J

Pediatric Defibrillation

- Rare occurrence; most pediatric codes are brady-asystolic
- Inadequate oxygenation is the most common cause of cardiac arrest in this age group
- Energy level is **2 J/kg** for initial countershock
- Double this level (**4 J/kg**) if unsuccessful and repeat × 2

Weight of Child	Initial shock
10 kg	20 J
20 kg	40 J
30 kg	60 J

Synchronized Cardioversion

Synchronized cardioversion is a distinct procedure that is not synonymous with unsynchronized defibrillation (countershock) and it specifically refers to the delivery of energy (in 4 to 30 msec) at a specific point in the cardiac cycle. It is used for **VT with a pulse that is unstable** and has not responded to medications and to a variety of **supraventricular tachycardias** (SVT) (e.g., atrial flutter, paroxysmal SVT, atrial fibrillation). The defibrillator senses the R wave of the ECG cycle to deliver the current, avoiding the T wave, which is the vulnerable period of the ECG cycle and, if delivered at this point, could put the patient into VF.

To accomplish this, you place the defibrillator in synchronous mode, (push a button or turn a switch—know your equipment). A marker usually shows up on the screen to indicate that you are synchronized. The defibrillator will deliver the energy when it senses it is appropriate after you push the buttons. You push and hold both buttons and wait for the defibrillator to fire. You are, in a sense, arming the defibrillator. It will decide when to fire.

Tachycardias with serious signs and symptoms directly related to the tachycardia can respond to cardioversion. Consider **premedication** of the patient whenever possible prior to cardioversion. Effective regimens have included diazepam, midazolam, barbiturates, etomidate, ketamine, and methohexital with or without an accompanying analgesic agent (e.g., fentanyl, morphine, meperidine). If the cardioverter is inexperienced with sedation techniques, it may be necessary to call anesthesia to assist with this aspect of the procedure.

Suggested energy levels for cardioversion are the following:

VT with pulse	100 J, 200 J, 300 J, 360 J
VT (polymorphic with irregular form and rate)	200 J, 200 J to 300 J, 360 J
Atrial fibrillation	100 J, 200 J, 300 J, 360 J
Atrial flutter	50 J, 100 J, 200 J, 300 J
SVTs (unresponsive to pharmacological treatment)	50 J, 100 J, 200 J, 300 J

Three key points to remember:

1. Most defibrillators will automatically reset to **unsynchronized defibrillation** mode after each synchronized cardioversion attempt. **Always** reset the machine for repeated cardioversions!
2. If the rate is very rapid (usually > 200 beats/min) and the QRS complex is very wide, the machine may deliver the energy during a vulnerable period and cause VF to result. **Always** have a full crash cart standing by for this potential complication. The initial energy level to use for VF in this setting is 200 J.
3. Cardioversion in the presence of digoxin toxicity is to be avoided![1] Cardioversion in the presence of therapeutic digoxin levels is now thought to be safe.[2]

The AHA algorithm for the treatment of tachycardia is found in Figure 9.1.

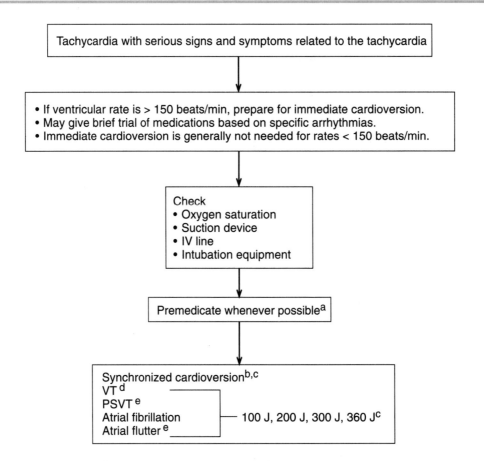

Tachycardia with serious signs and symptoms related to the tachycardia

- If ventricular rate is > 150 beats/min, prepare for immediate cardioversion.
- May give brief trial of medications based on specific arrhythmias.
- Immediate cardioversion is generally not needed for rates < 150 beats/min.

Check
- Oxygen saturation
- Suction device
- IV line
- Intubation equipment

Premedicate whenever possible[a]

Synchronized cardioversion[b,c]
VT [d]
PSVT [e]
Atrial fibrillation   100 J, 200 J, 300 J, 360 J[c]
Atrial flutter [e]

[a] Effective regimens have included a sedative (e.g., **diazepam, midazolam, barbiturates, etomidate, ketamine, methohexital**) with or without an analgesic agent (e.g., **fentanyl, morphine, meperidine**). Many experts recommend anesthesia if service is readily available.

[b] Note possible need to resynchronize after each cardioversion.

[c] If delays in synchronization occur and clinical conditions are critical, go to immediate unsynchronized shocks.

[d] Treat polymorphic VT (irregular form and rate) like VF: 200 J, 200–300 J, 360 J.

[e] PSVT and atrial flutter often respond to lower energy levels (start with 50 J).

■ **Figure 9.1**   Electrical cardioversion algorithm (with the patient not in cardiac arrest). Reproduced with permission. CPR Issue, JAMA, October 28, 1992. © American Heart Association.

Automatic Implantable Cardioverter-Defibrillators

Automatic implantable cardioverter-defibrillators (AICDs) are relatively new and are implanted in the patient's abdomen with wires leading to the myocardium. They are quite useful in those patients with repeated episodes of VT or VF that can prove fatal if not immediately treated.

Characteristics

- Wires lead from unit to three electrodes on the myocardium
- Senses rate only *or* rate plus wave form
- Fires three to seven times depending on setting
- Resets after a period of normal rhythm, then available to deliver another series
- Approximately 50 J delivered to myocardium
- If you are in contact with patient, you may feel small shock (not harmful)
- Do not withhold conventional defibrillation to wait for AICD to shock
- Internal AICD will not fire again until reset by regular rhythm
- Older design of electrode "patches" may interfere with external defibrillation

Pacing

The 1992 recommendations place more emphasis on transcutaneous rather than transvenous pacemakers in emergency situations. This is in great part due to the ease with which we can now pace patients. The most common indications for pacing are:

- Hemodynamically or symptomatically significant bradycardias (e.g., AV blocks, marked sinus bradycardias)
- Overdrive pacing of refractory tachycardias
- Prophylactic pacing in acute MIs with impaired conduction (e.g., Mobitz II, third-degree heart block)

The three types of pacers available include

1. Transcutaneous (external)
2. Transthoracic
3. Transvenous

External pacemakers are only a temporizing measure and may need to be replaced with a transvenous or permanent pacer later on. Pacing is also ineffective for pulseless electrical activity (PEA; previously called EMD), as electrical activity is present and pacing will not improve the underlying problem.

Many of the newer defibrillators include a built-in transcutaneous pacemaker, which greatly decreases the time required to commence cardiac pacing when indicated by the code situation. In your ACLS courses, if you have the opportunity to practice with such a defibrillator/pacer, it will be well worth the time.

Transvenous pacing is ideally used when fluoroscopy is available if ECG-guided placement is unsuccessful. It is usually inserted through either the brachial, subclavian, internal jugular, or femoral vein. If transvenous pacing is required by the clinical situation, transcutaneous pacing can be used to temporarily stabilize the patient.

Key Points

- Pacing is of no benefit with dead myocardial tissue (e.g., asystole resulting from a long code).
- Electrical capture *does not* mean a pulse will result.
- Muscular artifact *does not* mean pacing is occurring.
- The only criteria to determine successful pacing is a **pulse.**

- For permanent pacemakers, defibrillation paddles could be no closer than 5 inches from the battery pack.

Table 9.1 gives the AHA indications for emergent and standby pacing.

■ **Table 9.1**   **Indications for Emergent and Standby Pacing**

Emergent pacing

Hemodynamically compromising bradycardias[a]

(BP<80 mm Hg systolic, change in mental status, myocardial ischemia, pulmonary edema)

Bradycardia with malignant escape rhythms
(unresponsive to pharmacologic therapy)

Overdrive pacing of refractory tachycardia

Supraventricular or ventricular (currently indicated only in special situations refractory to pharmacologic therapy or cardioversion)

Bradyasystolic cardiac arrest

Pacing not routinely recommended in such patients. If used at all, pacing should be used as early as possible after onset of arrest.

Standby pacing

Stable bradycardias

(BP >80 mm Hg, no evidence of hemodynamic compromise, or hemodynamic compromise responsive to initial drug therapy)

Prophylactic pacing in acute myocardial infarction

Symptomatic sinus node dysfunction

Mobitz II second-degree heart block

Third-degree heart block

Newly acquired: left bundle-branch block, right bundle-branch block, alternating bundle-branch block, or bifascicular block

[a] Include complete heart block, symptomatic second-degree heart block, symptomatic sick sinus syndrome, drug-induced bradycardias (i.e., digoxin, ß-blockers, calcium channel blockers, or procainamide), permanent pacemaker failure, idioventricular bradycardias, symptomatic atrial fibrillation with slow ventricular response, refractory bradycardia during resuscitation of hypovolemic shock, and bradyarrhythmias with malignant ventricular escape mechanisms.

Reproduced with permission. CPR Issue, JAMA, October 28, 1992. © American Heart Association.

Automated External Defribillators and Semiautomated External Defribrillators

Automated external defibrillators (AEDs) and semiautomated external defibrillators (SAEDs) have been designed to aid non-ACLS personnel in delivering early defibrillation without extensive training (e.g., firemen, policemen). They are specifically *not* used by ACLS-trained personnel, as the information they give and the limited flexibility on treatment of arrhythmias makes them less than ideal for trained ACLS personnel.

Characteristics

- Utilizes algorithm-based internal software to diagnose shockable rhythms and deliver a shock
- Has achieved a high success rate and good safety record in the field
- Can **only** "diagnose" and treat VF or VT > 180 beats/min
- Should **never** be used for monitoring (limited rhythm detection ability and usually has no monitor screen!) unless you have an advanced model capable of carrying out this task
- If screen available with unit, usually *not* of good diagnostic quality
- Always check pulses on patients treated with an AED
- If the first responder using the AED has started the defibrillation process, let him or her finish. He or she can deliver the shocks faster than you can get your ACLS equipment hooked up.
- The shocks that are delivered by non-ACLS personnel (first responders) are "your" shocks; you have essentially delegated the "shocking" to them. Therefore, if they have delivered three shocks to the patient, you should continue on with the code process, (IV, epinephrine, ventilation, etc).
- While the machine is in the diagnostic mode, **do not** touch the patient. Do not perform CPR between shocks, as the machine cannot diagnose artifact and will default to the "no-shock" mode.

Steps for Operation of All AEDs

1. Turn on power.
2. Attach device to patient—modified lead II (upper-right sternal border and left midaxillary line over apex of heart).
3. Initiate analysis.
   A. AEDs take multiple "looks" at patient's rhythm
   B. **Must** stop CPR during analysis portion
4. Deliver shock, if indicated (make sure **all personnel clear!**)
   A. Average of 10 s to 15 s from activating analysis to delivery of actual shock to patient
   B. Experience reveals AEDs *not* misled by patient movement, transportation, or artifactual signals
   C. However, it is recommended not to place AED in *analysis mode* during patient or vehicle transport, as it may interfere with accurate rhythm assessment

Summary

Rapid defibrillation remains the major determinant of survival in cardiac arrest due to VF. Proper use of defibrillation and cardioversion is critical for the health care provider to fully understand and be comfortable with. During your ACLS course, take the time to become familiar with the various models available and learn not only how to charge and administer defibrillation and cardioversion but also how to troubleshoot common problems that may arise during use of the machine.

References

1. Lown B, DeSilva RA. The technique of cardioversion. In Hurts JW, ed. *The heart.* New York: McGraw-Hill, 1982, pp. 1752–1756.
2. Mann DL, Maisel AS, et al. Absence of cardioversion-induced ventricular arrhythmias in patients with therapeutic digoxin levels. *J Am Coll Cardiol* 1985;5:882–888.

Notes

10 Emergency Treatment of Cardiac Arrest

And as it is appointed unto men once to die, but after this the judgment"[1]

Objectives

1. Identify the need for providing early defibrillation in cardiac arrest.
2. Recognize the need for early advanced airway management.
3. Appreciate the magnitude of the problem of sudden cardiac death.
4. Recognize when it is appropriate to withhold, start, and discontinue resuscitative attempts.
5. Recognize the potential need for Critical Incident Stress Debriefing after an unsuccessful resuscitation attempt.

Sudden Cardiac Death

Good News and Bad News

The good news is that death from cardiovascular disease has declined during the past several decades.[2,3] The bad news is that despite improvements in diet, lifestyle, advancement in diagnostic capability, pharmacotherapy, and surgical interventions, cardiovascular disease still kills nearly one million Americans each year, and accounts for nearly half of the deaths from all causes in the United States. Coronary artery disease is responsible for approximately 500,000 deaths each year. The majority of these are due to sudden death.[4] What makes this problem even more vexing is that two thirds of all sudden deaths occur outside the hospital setting, usually within two hours of the onset of symptoms.[2, 5–10].

Sudden death due to CAD has become the most prominent medical emergency in the United States today.[11] In addition to being the most prominent, it is also the most inconvenient. It happens in the worst possible setting (out-of-hospital) and can occur without warning. In fact, the majority of patients who experience sudden death have no warning symptoms at all immediately prior to collapse. Indeed, sudden death may be the first manifestation of underlying heart disease in up to 20% of patients.[12–14]

Approximately 80% to 90% of adults with sudden, nontraumatic cardiac arrest are found to be in VF when the initial ECG is obtained.[15] While electrical defibrillation is the most effective means of reversing VF,[16, 17] its success is most dependent on how quickly it can be administered.[16,18–20] Patients experiencing primary VF occurring in a coronary care unit or with a witnessed cardiac arrest occurring in a cardiac rehabilitation center can almost always be successfully resuscitated.[21]

The successful resuscitation rates from VF in these settings have prompted the recommendation that the community be viewed as the "ultimate Coronary Care Unit."[22] All too often, however, if witnesses to a cardiac arrest are present, they are unprepared to deal with it.

Key Points

- Sudden cardiac death is the most prominent medical emergency in the United States today.
- Ventricular fibrillation is the most commonly occurring rhythm disturbance in the adult, nontraumatic cardiac arrest patient.
- Gloves and a face mask are important adjuncts to bystander CPR.
- Defibrillation should be performed as soon as possible.
- Early EMS access is critical to the resuscitation process.
- Endotracheal intubation should be performed as soon as is practical.

- Unsuccessful field ACLS warrants discontinuation of efforts and nontransportation to the emergency department.
- Serious psychological disturbances may occur after an unsuccessful resuscitation attempt.

Preparing for Sudden Death

Witnesses to sudden death can control neither the location nor the timing of the event. Preparation is the one variable that can be controlled.

Most health-care providers are prepared to deal with an emergency situation in the context of their professional setting and, by definition, are obligated to do so. Fortunately, most, if not all, medical settings will have the personnel and equipment available to respond to a sudden cardiac event. The environment has been prepared to handle such a contingency. However, since most sudden deaths occur outside a controlled medical environment, anyone inclined to become involved in an out-of-hospital emergency should likewise be prepared.

Psychological Preparation

All medical professionals need to consider whether they would be willing to become involved if an emergency arises outside of the workplace. How involved would you become? Are you willing to initiate the call for help? Are you prepared psychologically to respond as a bystander and perform basic life support? Are you willing to become involved physically by providing CPR? How would you react if the victim were a friend or a relative? Could you function in such a circumstance?

Unless you provide emergency medical care on a routine basis, if you answer honestly, you probably cannot predict how you would respond to a medical emergency in an unusual setting. One way of preparing, mentally, is to try to visualize yourself in such a situation. Picture the most unlikely place to be recruited into action. See the face of an unconscious stranger. Consider what your reaction to a pool of blood, vomitus, or excrement would be. Now imagine that you are the only trained person there. Assuming you want to act, could you?

Physical Preparation

Having mentally rehearsed your performance as a bystander to an emergency event, you determine that you would and could function under such conditions. Are you equipped physically to perform the tasks required of you?

Given the time that we live in, the concept of universal precautions should extend to include the out-of-hospital setting. Everyone, from law enforcement personnel to boxing referees, is beginning to wear gloves when the potential for coming into contact with bodily fluids exists. If there is the remotest possibility that you may become involved in an out-of-hospital emergency, a little foresight and preparation could provide future peace of mind. There is a saying, "if it's warm and wet and it isn't yours, wear gloves."

The empty plastic container from a 35-mm roll of film becomes a small and effective receptacle for a pair of surgical gloves, keeping them fresh until needed. Many firefighters have begun to keep a pair of gloves ready like this in the pocket of their turnout coats.

Commercial airway barriers are available for use by the health care provider and lay public. Some are small enough to be carried on a key chain. The convenient size is offset by the need to actively adjust the barrier to allow exhalation. Larger, more effective face masks are available that have a one-way valve so that the rescuer need not be exposed to the patient's expired air. Some of these also have a head strap to help maintain position and have a port for an oxygen supply to be attached. These larger masks are still small enough to be carried in a pocket or purse.

Dealing with Sudden Death

Assessment

Previously, if a patient were found to be in cardiac arrest, it was recommended that CPR be initiated for one minute prior to seeking assistance. However, because of the critical need to provide defibrillation as soon as possible, it is now recommended that the EMS system be activated once unresponsiveness is determined.[11] If two rescuers are present, one should access the EMS system while the other continues basic life support.

Treatment

There is no doubt that early defibrillation for the treatment of out-of-hospital cardiac arrest due to VF is effective in saving lives. As such, defibrillation is classified by the AHA as a Class 1 intervention ("usually indicated, always acceptable, and considered useful and effective"). With early defibrillation programs, survival to hospital discharge with full recovery can be as high as 30% for some victims of sudden cardiac arrest.[22]

Early defibrillation is now considered the highest priority in cardiac arrest. The AHA considers early defibrillation to be the standard of care in the community.[23] The 1992 National Conference on Cardiopulmonary Resuscitation and Emergency Cardiac Care has called for all personnel whose jobs require that they perform basic CPR to be trained to operate and be permitted to use defibrillators. With the availability of AEDs today, defibrillation can be considered part of basic life support. Failure of emergency personnel to have a defibrillator during a cardiac arrest may be difficult to defend.[11]

Defibrillation is the single most important intervention in adult emergency cardiac care. It must be remembered that defibrillation is ineffective without an adequate airway and effective ventilation.[11] Although defibrillation has become an accepted part of basic life support, definitive, advanced airway management (i.e., ET intubation) has unfortunately remained within the realm of advanced life support.

In an attempt to remedy this, ET intubation, a Class 1 intervention, has been moved further up in the algorithm for the treatment of cardiac arrest. It is now recommended that the trachea be intubated "as soon as is practical during the resuscitative effort."[11]

Once the EMS system has been activated, while awaiting the arrival of a defibrillator, the bystander can hope to buy some time by performing basic life support. Bystander CPR is the best treatment that a cardiac arrest patient can receive until the arrival of a defibrillator and ACLS care.[24,25] Although bystander CPR is clearly of value, it is only temporizing and loses its value if early defibrillation and ACLS do not rapidly follow.[11]

Initiating Cardiopulmonary Resuscitation

Because it is impossible to reliably determine potential brain viability at the onset of cardiac arrest, the anticipated neurologic status should *not* be used as criteria for determining whether to begin CPR. Rather, cardiovascular unresponsiveness is the sole criteria used for determining the need for a resuscitation attempt. Given this, if CPR is begun based on cardiovascular unresponsiveness, the presumption of potential brain viability has been made.

In the hospital setting, absent a formal "do not resuscitate" (DNR) document, it is presumed that resuscitation for a victim of cardiac or respiratory arrest will be provided.[11] In the out-of-hospital setting, unless you are a member of a formal EMS team, it is unlikely that you will have to deal with a written DNR form. It is possible, but improbable, that a person would be up and about in the community with such a document on their person.

It is recognized that in some circumstances it may be appropriate *not* to initiate CPR. Such conditions include the presence of obvious clinical signs of death, cases where attempts at resuscitation would place the health care provider at significant risk of physical injury, or cases where there is documentation or another reliable reason to believe that CPR is not indicated, wanted, or in the person's best interest.

Unwitnessed deaths in the presence of known serious, chronic, debilitating disease or in the terminal state of a fatal illness may be a reliable criterion in some settings to believe that CPR is not indicated.[11]

In some instances it may be difficult to determine if cardiac resuscitation should be initiated. On occasion, even when a DNR order is present, a family member may request that CPR be performed. If there is reasonable doubt that the "no-CPR order" is invalid, CPR should be performed.

Accepting the Inevitable

In a study of 3,221 victims of nontraumatic, out-of-hospital cardiac arrest in Chicago, only 2% survived to be discharged from the hospital. The survival rate for those presenting in VF was only 3%.[26]

Some EMS systems require that all cardiac arrest patients in whom a resuscitation attempt is begun be transported to the hospital. Other systems routinely terminate unsuccessful CPR efforts in the field.[11] Several studies have demonstrated the futility of transporting a patient to the emergency department if spontaneous circulation has not been restored after adequate ACLS has been performed in the field.[27-29]

Since 1973, over 50 million people have learned CPR.[11] Although CPR is considered a successful public health initiative, the average survival rate to hospital discharge is only 15%, although some studies have reported a favorable neurologic status among such survivors.[30] This means that, in more than four out of five times, rescuers trained to save lives were unsuccessful.[11]

Health care providers must realize ahead of time that not everyone will "be saved." Accepting this as part of life can help avoid side effects after an unsuccessful resuscitation attempt is encountered.

Serious long-lasting physical and emotional symptoms may occur in health care providers who attempt unsuccessful CPR. They may actually go through a grief reaction and experience chronic anxiety, depression, and burnout.[11]

In order to avoid such reactions, it is recommended that anyone involved in an unsuccessful CPR attempt be offered the option of receiving a Critical Incident Stress Debriefing in order to confront and discuss his or her thoughts and feelings relative to the call. This is especially important when the incident has more potential for trauma, such as when a child or multiple victims are involved.

Postponing the Inevitable

Although not all patients survive, you can help improve a patient's chances of being able to survive an out-of-hospital cardiac arrest. Those that are most likely to be present at the scene of an out-of-hospital cardiac arrest should be encouraged to learn CPR. This includes family members of patients with known cardiac disease, especially those with a history of already surviving an out-of-hospital cardiac arrest. Senior citizens, likewise, are an ideal population to reach out to in providing training in CPR.

Wishful Thinking

Does your community have a rapid defibrillation program? If you do not know, find out. If it does not, find out why not. What is the recommended emergency access telephone number in your area? Is it posted on your telephone? Do your children know how to call for help? Do you have your house numbers visible and/or lighted, so that an ambulance can easily locate your house?

Summary

This chapter has highlighted some of the critical points in dealing with the treatment of sudden death. An excellent review article by Myerburg et al.[31] on the epidemiology, risk, and intervention assessment covers this topic in more depth. ACLS training provides you with the tools needed to maximize your ability to save lives. Remember to be prepared.

References

1. The King James Bible. Hebrews 9:27.
2. American Heart Association. 1992 Heart and stroke facts. Dallas, Tex.: American Heart Association, 1991.
3. Goldman L, Cook EF. The decline in ischemic heart disease mortality rates: An analysis of the comparative effects of medical interventions and changes in lifestyle. *Ann Intern Med* 1984;101:825–836.
4. *Morbidity and mortality chartbook on cardiovascular, lung and blood diseases 1990*. Bethesda, Md.: National Heart, Lung, and Blood Institute: 1990.
5. Bainton CR, Peterson DR. Deaths from coronary heart disease in persons 50 years of age and younger: A community-wide study. *N Engl J Med* 1963;268:569–575.
6. Kuller L, Lilienfeld A, Flusher R. Sudden and unexpected deaths in young adults: An epidemiological study. *JAMA* 1966;198:248–252.
7. Kuller L, Lilienfeld A, Flusher R. Epidemiological study of sudden and unexpected deaths due to arteriosclerotic heart disease. *Circulation* 1966; 34:1056–1068.
8. McNeilly RAH, Pemberton J. Duration of last attack in 998 fatal cases of coronary artery disease and its relation to possible cardiac resuscitation. *Br Med J* 1968;3:139–142.
9. Gordon T, Kannel WB. Premature mortality from coronary heart disease: The Framingham study. *JAMA* 1971;215:1617–1625.
10. Carveth SW. Eight year experience with a stadium-based mobile coronary care unit. *Heart Lung* 1974;3:770–774.
11. American Heart Association. Guidelines for cardiopulmonary resuscitation and emergency cardiac care. *JAMA* 1992;268:2171–2302.
12. Schaffer WA, Cobb LA. Recurrent ventricular fibrillation and modes of death in survivors of out-of-hospital ventricular fibrillation. *N Engl J Med* 1975;293:259–262.
13. Baum RS, Alvarez H 3rd, Cobb LA. Survival after resuscitation from out-of-hospital ventricular fibrillation. *Circulation* 1974;50:1231–1235.
14. Eisenberg MS, Cummins RO, Litwin PE, et al. Out-of-hospital cardiac arrest: Significance of symptoms in patients collapsing before and after arrival of paramedics. *Am J Emerg Med* 1986;4:116–120.
15. Bayes de Luna A, Coumel P, Loclerq JF. Ambulatory sudden cardiac death: Mechanisms of production of fatal arrhythmia on the basis of data from 157 cases. *Am Heart J* 1989;117:151–159.

16. Eisenberg MS, Copass MK, Hallstrom AP, et al. Treatment of out-of-hospital cardiac arrests with rapid defibrillation by emergency medical technicians. *N Engl J Med* 1980;302:1379–1383.
17. Stults KR, Brown DD, Schug VL, et al. Prehospital defibrillation performed by emergency medical technicians in rural communities. *N Engl J Med* 1984;310:219–223.
18. Eisenberg MA, Bergner L, Hallstrom AP. Paramedic programs and out-of-hospital cardiac arrest: Factors associated with successful resuscitation. *Am J Publ Health* 1979;69:30–38.
19. Cobb LA, Hallstrom AP. Community-based cardiopulmonary resuscitation: What have we learned? *Ann NY Acad Sci* 1982;382:330–342.
20. Weaver WD, Copass MK, Buffi D, et al. Improved neurologic recovery and survival after early defibrillation. *Circulation* 1984;69:943–948.
21. Hossack KF, Hartwig R. Cardiac arrest associated with supervised cardiac rehabilitation. *J Cardiac Rehab* 1982;2:402.
22. Cobb LA. Prehospital cardiac care: Does it make a difference? *Am Heart J* 1982;103:316–318.
23. Kerber RE. Statement on early defibrillation from the Emergency Cardiac Care Committee, American Heart Association. *Circulation* 1991;83:2233.
24. Standards and guidelines for cardiopulmonary resuscitation (CPR) and emergency cardiac care (ECC), part VII: Emergency cardiac care units (in EMS systems). *JAMA* 1986;225:2974–2979.
25. Putting it all together: Resuscitation of the patient. In: Jaffe A, ed. *Textbook of advanced cardiac life support*, 1987. Dallas, Tex.: American Heart Association, 1987; pp. 235–248.
26. Becker LB, Ostrander MP, Barrett J, et al. CPR Chicago. Outcome of CPR in a large metropolitan area—where are the survivors? *Ann Emerg Med* 1991;20:355–361.
27. Kellerman AL, Staves, DR, Hackman, BB. In-hospital resuscitation following unsuccessful prehospital advanced cardiac life support: "Heroic efforts" or an exercise in futility? *Ann Emerg Med.* 1988;17:589–594.
28. Gray WA, Capone KJ, Most AS. Unsuccessful emergency medical resuscitation: Are continued efforts in the emergency department justified? *N Engl J Med* 1991;325:1393–1398.
29. Bonnin MJ, Popo PE, Clark PS. Key role of prehospital resuscitation in survival from out-of-hospital cardiac arrest. *Ann Emerg Med* 1990;19:466. Abstract.
30. Simmons ML, Kimman GP, Ivens EMA, et al. Follow up after out of hospital resuscitation. Read before the XIIth Annual Congress of the European Society of Cardiology. Stockholm, Sweden: September 16–20, 1990.
31. Myerburg RJ, Kessler KM, Castellanos A. Sudden cardiac death: Epidemiology, transient risk and intervention assessment. *Ann Intern Med* 1993;119:1187–1197.

11 Essential Drugs for Adult Resuscitations

Objectives

1. Recognize the changes in recommended pharmacologic agents for use in resuscitation.
2. State the correct dosages and intervals for recommended medications used during resuscitations.
3. List medications with their appropriate dosages that may be administered via an ET tube.
4. Identify recommendations concerning the IV administration of medications.

Overview

The new protocols and recommendations from the ECC of the AHA have made some major changes to some of the medication regimens of 1986. This chapter summarizes the major changes you will encounter in the new ACLS course.

Key Points

- *Epinephrine* (cardiac arrest dose) is 1.0 mg by IV push and should be repeated every 3 to 5 min. Epinephrine via continuous IV infusion will be used more frequently in place of isoproterenol as a temporizing measure for significant bradycardia.

- **Atropine** is only expected to be effective when the block is at the AV node or higher or when there is a significant vagal component to the bradydysrhythmias. It is less useful in idioventricular rhythms, Mobitz II, third-degree AV block, and asystole. Some patients may require 3.0 mg of atropine to achieve a full vagolytic dose.
- **Procainamide's** new recommended loading dose is 17 mg/kg (rather than the old dosage of 1,000 mg). This should be given no faster than 20 to 30 mg/min while monitoring the blood pressure, pulse, QRS duration, and QT interval.
- **Adenosine** is recommended for use with PSVT but is **not** indicated for atrial fibrillation or atrial flutter.
- **Verapamil** may be used for the treatment of narrow-complex PSVT following adenosine. In atrial fibrillation and atrial flutter, however, verapamil will only *slow* the ventricular response *but will not break* these rhythms. In general, **do not** use for wide-complex tachycardias. It is also contraindicated in VT, Wolff-Parkinson-White syndrome, and usually in PSVT with aberrancy.
- **Diltiazem** in its IV form is now considered a core drug for atrial fibrillation, atrial flutter, and PSVT as well. The dose is 0.25 mg/kg initially over 1 to 2 minutes in adults. A repeat dose may be given in 15 minutes. If indicated, this may be followed by a continuous IV drip at 5 to 15 mg/hr.
- **Magnesium** is the drug of choice in the treatment of Torsades de Pointes and is optional in the ventricular algorithm.
- **Isoproterenol** is *no longer* recommended for emergency cardiac care. It has a very narrow margin of safety, and increased myocardial oxygen consumption results from its use. If a catecholamine drip is required as a temporizing measure, the guidelines recommend either a dopamine or epinephrine infusion.

Several medications can be given down the ET tube when venous access to the central circulation is not possible. These include the following (adult doses):

Narcan	N	Usual dose of 0.4–2.0 mg
Epinephrine	E	2 to 2.5 times peripheral dose
Atropine	A	Double the usual dose
Lidocaine	L	Double the usual dose

Remember, medications may require a reduction in dosage for patients who are elderly, who have impaired liver or renal function, or who receive an infusion for greater than 24 hours. It is imperative that all medication administration be monitored consistently and that the lowest *therapeutically effective* dose possible be used.

During the ACLS course, you will be expected to be familiar with about 23 different medications. Studying them thoroughly before attending the course will improve your ability to concentrate on practicing their proper administration rather than trying to learn their basic physiologic properties.

High-dose epinephrine (5 mg or 0.1 mg/kg) is *only* acceptable when conventional levels have failed to produce a clinical response. A study comparing standard-dose and high-dose epinephrine in cardiac arrest outside the hospital failed to demonstrate any difference in the overall rate of return of spontaneous circulation, survival to hospital admission, survival to hospital discharge, or neurologic outcome.[1] The AHA states that high-dose epinephrine should either be used or discussed for those who fail to respond to the standard doses.

Table 11.1 on page 114 lists usage, dosage, and potential complications for medications commonly utilized during arrest situations and about which you must be knowledgeable for the ACLS course.[2]

References

1. Brown CG, Martin DR, Pepe PE, et al. A comparison of standard-dose and high-dose epinephrine in cardiac arrest outside the hospital. *NEJM* 1992; 327:1051–1055.
2. American Heart Association. Guidelines for Cardiopulmonary Resuscitation and Emergency Cardiac Care. *JAMA* 1992;268:2171–2302.

■ **Table 11.1**   **ACLS Drug Chart**

Drug	Use	Dosage	Complications
Adenosine Supplied: 3 mg/mL in 2-mL vials (total = 6 mg)	PSVTs (involving re-entry pathway including AV node)	6 mg rapid IV bolus over 1 s to 3 s. Follow with 20 mL saline flush Repeat with 12-mg rapid IV push if no response within 1 to 2 min	Avoid in second- or third-degree heart block and sick sinus syndrome Dyspnea, flushing, chest pain (all side effects usually resolve within 1 to 2 min) Transient sinus bradycardia or ventricular ectopy may occur after terminating SVT Dipyridamole potentiates its effects Theophylline decreases effects
Amrinone Supplied: 5 mg/mL in 20-mL vials (total =100 mg). Mix in 0.45% normal saline to maximum of 3 mg/mL (750mg/ 250 mL)	1. Low cardiac output 2. Refractory CHF	Loading dose: 0.75 mg/kg over 2 to 3 min, followed by infusion of 5 to 15 µg/kg/ min	Worsen ventricular ectopy Exacerbate myocardial ischemia
Atropine Supplied: 0.1 mg/ mL in 10-mL preloaded syringes (total =1 mg) Can be given via ET tube	1. Sinus bradycardia 2. Asystole 3. AV block at nodal level	Asystole and slow PEA: 1 mg IV and repeat in 3 to 5 min Bradycardia: 0.5 mg to 1.0 mg IV every 3 to 5 min to a total dose of 0.04 mg/kg (= 3 mg*)	Increases myocardial oxygen demands Can increase ischemia or infarction (secondary to excessive increase in rate) Avoid in glaucoma Rare VF/VT with IV use Can trigger tachyarrhythmias and angina *Reserve total vagolytic dose of 3 mg for asystolic arrest

Drug	Use	Dosage	Complications
β-adrenergic blockers Supplied: *Metoprolol:* 1 mg/mL in 5 = mL vials (total = 5 mg). *Atenolol:* 0.5 mg/mL in 10-mL ampules (total = 5 mg) *Propranolol:* 4 mg/mL in 5-mL vials (total = 20 mg)	1. Thrombolytic treated patients (may reduce reinfarction rate and ischemia) 2. Prevent VF in post-MI patients 3. Stable angina	*Atenolol:* 5 mg to 10 mg IV over 5 min *Metoprolol:* 5 mg to 10 mg slow IV push at 5-min intervals until total of 15 mg. *Oral:* 50 mg BID to 100 mg BID after 24 hrs *Propranolol:* total dose of 0.1mg/kg by slow IV push in 3 equal doses at 2 to 3-min intervals (do not exceed rate of 1 mg/min). *Oral:* 180 mg/day to 320 mg/day in divided doses	Hypotension AV conduction delays Bradycardias Decreased myocardial contraction Avoid in patients with asthma/COPD, diabetes, PVD
Bretylium Supplied: 50 mg/mL in 10-mL prefilled syringes (total = 500 mg); 50 mg/mL in 10 = mL vials (total = 500 mg	1. VF and VT after defibrillation, epinephrine, and lidocaine have failed 2. Wide-complex tachycardias unresponsive to lidocaine and adenosine	VF: 5 mg/kg IV bolus. If VF persists, increase to 10 mg/kg and repeat every 5 min up to maximum of 30 mg/kg to 35 mg/kg Recurrent VT: 5 mg/kg to 10 mg/kg diluted in 50 mL D5W IV over 8 to 10 min Infusion: 1 mg/min to 2 mg/min (mix 500 mg in 250 mL of D5W)	Hypotension Bradycardia Nausea and vomiting with rapid IV administration Dizziness/syncope Do not use in known aortic stenosis Use with extreme caution in arrhythmias due to digitalis toxicity
Calcium Supplied: 100 mg/mL in 10 = mL vials (total = 1gm; a 10% solution)	1. Hypocalcemia 2. Calcium channel blocker toxicity 3. Hyperkalemia	10% solution of CaCl in a dose of 2 mg/kg to 4 mg/kg and repeated as necessary at 10-min intervals Ca gluconate in a dose of 5 mL to 8 mL	Hypercalcemia Arrhythmias (e.g., bradycardia, asystole, VF) Extravasation may cause tissue necrosis

Drug	Use	Dosage	Complications
Digitalis Supplied: 0.5mg/2 mL 0.1mg/1mL	1. Atrial arrhythmias 2. CHF	Loading dose: 0.5 mg IV or po, followed by 0.25 mg IV/po Q 6H (total dose = 1 mg) For acute suppression of atrial arrhythmias, drug can be given 0.25 mg IV Q 30 to 45 min	AV block Bradycardia Arrhythmias Monitor blood levels Avoid hypokalemia
Dobutamine Supplied: 12.5 mg/mL in 20-mL vials (total = 250 mg)	1. Low cardiac output 2. Treatment of heart failure 3. Increase myocardial contractility	Infusion: 2 to 20 µg/kg/min Infusion: Dilute 500 mg to 1,000 mg (40 mL to 80 mL) in 250 mL NS or D5W	Increased heart rate, which may exacerbate ischemia and can cause angina and increased BP PVCs Reflex peripheral vasodilation with secondary hypotension
Dopamine Supplied: 40 mg/mL in 5-mL ampules (total = 200 mg) or 160 mg/mL (total = 800 mg) IV infusion: mix 400 mg to 800 mg in 250 mL NS, LR, or D5W	1. Decreased urine output 2. Low cardiac output 3. Hypotension	Renal dose: 1 to 2 µg/kg/min Increased cardiac output: 2 to 10 µg/kg/min Hypotension: >10 µg/kg/min Infusion: 2.5 to 5 µg/kg/min and titrate to effect	Increased HR Arrhythmias Undesirable degree of vasoconstriction **Do not** use with bicarbonate in same IV line *or* in patients with hypotention secondary to hypovolemia MAO inhibitors potentiate effects of dopamine
Epinephrine Supplied: Preloaded 10-mL syringe: 1 mg/10 mL Glass 1-mL ampule: 1 mg/mL Multidose 30-mL vials: 1 mg/mL Can be given via ET tube	1. VF 2. Asystole 3. Symptomatic bradycardia (though not first-line agent)	1.0 mg (10 mL of 1:10,000 solution) IV every 3 to 5 min. Follow with 20 mL flush of IV fluid If this dose fails, 5 mg or 0.1 mg/kg (acceptable, but neither recommended nor discouraged)	Increased HR Arrhythmias Ischemia Do not administer in same line as alkaline solutions Peripheral injections should be followed by 20-mL flush of IV fluid

Drug	Use	Dosage	Complications
Epinephrine (con't)		Infusion: 1 mg (1 mL of 1:1,000 solution) added to 500 mL NS/ D5W and given 2 to 10 µg/min Endotracheal: 2 mg to 2.5 mg diluted in 10 mL NS	to assist with effective distribution of drug Administration for continuous infusions should be through central access to reduce extravasation
Furosemide Supplied: 10 mg/mL in ampules Syringes of 2 mL, 4 mL, 10 mL		0.5 mg/kg to 1.0 mg/ kg IV slowly *Oral:* 20 mg to 40 mg po initially, increase dose as clinically indicated	Hypotension Hyponatremia Dehydration Hypokalemia
Isoproterenol Supplied: 1 mg/mL in 1-mL vials IV infusion: Mix 1 mg in 250 mL NS, LR, or D5W	Significant bradycardia (temporary therapy only) Torsades de pointes	Infusion: 2 ug/min to 10 ug/min	Can exacerbate ischemia and arrhythmias (PVCs, VT) Increases cardiac output and myocardial work Not indicated in cardiac arrest or hypotension **Do not mix with epinephrine!**
IV fluids	1. Expand blood volume 2. Keep IV lines patent	IV lines: Normal saline or lactated Ringer's preferred, but may use D5W	Do not give fluids without indication of volume depletion Monitor for overload
Lidocaine Supplied: Preloaded 20 mg/mL in 5-mL syringes; also: 10 mg/mL in 5-mL vials in 5-mL vials (total = 50 mg) Can be given via ET tube	1. Ventricular ectopy (PVCs) 2. VF 3. VT 4. Wide-complex PSVT or tachyarrhythmias of uncertain type	Bolus: 1.0 mg/kg to 1.5 mg/kg with additional bolus of 0.5 mg/kg to 1.5 mg/kg every 5 to 10 min as needed until 3 mg/kg total Infusion: 2 mg/min to 4 mg/min (mix 1 gm in 500 mL of D5W)	Confusion Agitation Heart block Decrease dose after 24 hours or monitor levels Reduce second dose 50% in CHF, acute MI, liver failure, the elderly, and in patients with shock Do not use in bradycardiac-related PVCs

Drug	Use	Dosage	Complications
Magnesium sulfate Supplied: 10-mL ampules of 50% MgSO4 = 5 gm of magnesium; 2-mL ampules: (total = 1 gm/2 mL)	Magnesium deficiency, which is associated with cardiac arrhythmias	Load: 1 g to 2 g mixed in 50 mL to 100 mL of D5W and given over 5 to 60 min Infusion: 0.5 g to 1.0 g (4 mEq to 8 mEq) per hour for up to 24 hours	Monitor blood levels Drowsiness Respiratory depression
Morphine Supplied: 2 to 5 mg/mL in 1-mL syringes	1. Acute MI pain 2. Pulmonary edema	1 mg to 3 mg IV every 5 min as needed	Decreased respiratory drive Nausea and vomiting Hypotension Avoid use in head-injury patients
Nitroglycerin Supplied: SL tablets: 0.3, 0.4 mg Inhaler: 0.4 mg/dose Ampules: 5 mg in 10 mL 8 mg in 10 mL 10 mg in 10 mL	1. Angina 2. CHF associated with acute MI 3. Hypertension (IV use)	0.3 or 0.4 mg sublingually and repeat Q 3 to 5 min for a total of 3 tabs Infusion: 10 μg/min to 20 μg/min and increase by 5 μg/min to 10 μg/min Q 5 to 10 min (mix 50 or 100 mg in 250 mL D5W or saline)	Hypotension Headache Flushing Tachycardia Pardoxical bradyccardia Avoid use in glaucoma, hypotension, and suspected tamponade
Norepinephrine Supplied: 1 mg/mL in 4-mL ampules Mix 4 mg in 250 mL D5W or D5NS. Avoid diluting in NS alone.	1. Severe hypotension 2. Shock	Infusion: 0.5 μg/min to 1.0 μg/min Refractory shock: 8 ug/min to 30 μg/min	Increased vasoconstriction Severe headaches Increased myocardial oxygen consumption Do not administer in same line as alkaline solutions Relatively contraindicated in hypovolemic patients Administer through central access

Drug	Use	Dosage	Complications
Oxygen	1. Ischemia 2. Hypoxemia 3. Cardiac arrest	Highest concentration possible; 100% via ET tube	Rare: oxygen toxicity Use concentration of 24% to 35% in patients with COPD
Procainamide Supplied: 100 mg/mL in 10-mL vials (total = 8 g) 500 mg/mL in 2-mL vials (total = 1 g)	1. Suppression of PVCS and recurrent VT when lidocaine contra-indicated or failed 2. Acceptable for wide-complex tachycardias indistinguishable from VT	Infusion: 20 mg/min until: 1. 17 mg/kg total given 2. QRS widens more than 50% 3. Hypotension develops 4. Arrhythmia suppressed Maintenance: 1 mg/min to 4 mg/min (mix 1 g in 250 mL D5W)	QRS widening Hypotension AV block CNS depression Reduce dose and monitor levels in renal failure Avoid in patients with prolonged QT, digitalis toxicity, and torsades de pointes
Sodium bicarbonate Supplied: 50-mL preloaded syringe (8.4% sodium bicarbonate at 50 mEq/50 mL)	1. Metabolic acidosis 2. Beneficial in patients with pre-existing hyperkalemia	1 mEq/kg as initial dose, then half every 10 min Use ABGs to guide all therapy	Alkalosis Electrolyte abnormalities (e.g.,hypokalemia) Avoid use in hypokalemic patients
Sodium nitroprusside Supplied: 10 mg/mL in 5-mL vials (total = 50 mg)	1. Hypertension 2. Heart failure	Infusion: 0.1 to 5 µg/kg/min (mix 50 mg to 100 mg in 250 mL D5W) Light sensitive: Cover IV bag with opaque material	Hypotension, reflex tachycardia, angina Decrease dose in renal or liver failure Monitor for cyanide toxicity (blood levels)

Drug	Use	Dosage	Complications
Verapamil and Diltiazem Supplied: *Verapamil:* 2.5 mg/mL in 2-4-, and 5-mL vials (totals = 5, 10, and 12.5 mg) *Diltiazem:* 5 mg/mL in 5- or 10-mL vials (totals = 25 or 50 mg)	Control ventricular response in 1. Atrial flutter 2. Atrial fibrillation 3. Multifocal atrial tachycardia 4. Other SVTs 5. Narrow-complex PSVTs (Note: adenosine is drug of choice)	*Verapamil:* 2.5 mg to 5 mg IV over 2 min Repeat doses of 5 mg to 10 mg every 15 to 30 min to a maximum of 20 mg *Diltiazem:* 0.25 mg/kg followed by a second dose of 0.35 mg/kg In atrial fibrillation, infusion of 5 to 15 mg/ hr may be used	Decrease myocardial contractility in patients with LV dysfunction Exacerbate CHF in patients with LV dysfunction Hypotension AV block Nausea/vomiting

12 Don't Forget Those Special Resuscitation Situations

Stroke

Stroke is an illness of sudden onset caused by rupture or occlusion of a blood vessel, and approximately 75% are caused by ischemia (blood clot or embolism). Hemorrhagic stroke is the result of a ruptured cerebral blood vessel and can be fatal.[1]

Key Points

- The most important differential diagnosis to make is between *hemorrhagic* vs. *ischemic* stroke.
- Patients with subarachnoid hemorrhage may have an intense headache *without* any focal neurologic signs.
- Always ensure an adequate airway for stroke victims.
- Always monitor cardiac rhythm in patients with stroke to detect arrhythmias. In suspected cardiac sources, an echocardiogram and 24-hour Holter monitoring may be needed.
- Ocular hemorrhages may allow early identification of intracranial bleeding.
- The Glasgow Coma Scale[2] is used to assess the severity of neurologic damage.
- In comatose patients or those with C-spine tenderness/pain, a lateral C-spine x-ray should be performed to locate a fracture or dislocation.
- All computerized tomography (CT) testing should be without contrast enhancement as > 95% of all intracerebral bleeds and subarachnoid hemorrhages can be identified with nonenhanced CTs.
- Significant elevations of blood pressure (BP) (> 200 mm Hg systolic or 130 mm Hg calculated mean) after *ischemic* stroke should be treated cautiously as response to therapy may be exaggerated in this setting. Blood pressure may also decline spontaneously when agitation, vomiting, or pain is brought under control.
- Glucose IV can be given if hypoglycemia is suspected.
- Always rule out hypoglycemia in a *diabetic* patient presenting with an apparent acute stroke.
- Avoid rapid infusions of saline into patients with stroke unless significant hypotension is suspected or known (high infusions will tend to promote cerebral edema).
- Avoid using D5W as your infusion fluid (unless patient is truly hypoglycemic), as this is a hypotonic fluid that can increase cerebral edema.

Seizure Control

- Stroke patients may experience seizures. Treatment can be with **lorazepam** (1 to 2 mg IV) or **diazepam** (5 to 10 mg IV).

- Intravenous **phenytoin (Dilantin)** can be used to prevent *further* seizures given in a loading dose of 15 mg/kg. *Do not give faster than 50 mg/min to avoid any potential cardiac toxicity!*
- **Dexamethasone/steroids** are of unproven use in acute stroke and their routine administration is not indicated.
- No heparin should be given to any patient with acute or progressive ischemic stroke until a CT scan has ruled out the presence of an intracranial bleed.
- **Aspirin** and **warfarin** have *unproven* value in acute stroke (but may be useful in preventing strokes).
- Obtain neurological and neurosurgical consultations as indicated.

Table 12.1 shows the clinical representations of acute stroke. Table 12.2 lists the proper assessment of the patient with an acute stroke. Table 12.3 lists the initial laboratory and radiologic studies recommended for evaluation of a patient with an acute stroke. Table 12.4 shows the recommended emergency treatment for a stroke patient. Figure 12.1 shows the new AHA algorithm for the initial evaluation of suspected stroke.

■ **Table 12.1**   **Clinical Representations of Acute Stroke**

Alteration in consciousness (coma, stupor, confusion, seizures, delirium)
Intense or unusually severe headache of sudden onset or any headache associated with decreased level of consciousness or neurologic deficit, unusual and severe neck or facial pain
Aphasia (incoherent speech or difficulty understanding speech)
Facial weakness or asymmetry (paralysis of the facial muscles, usually noted when the patient speaks or smiles); may be on the same side or opposite side from limb paralysis
Incoordination, weakness, paralysis, or sensory loss of one or more limbs; usually involves one half of the body and in particular the hand
Ataxia (poor balance, clumsiness, or difficulty walking)
Visual loss (monocular or binocular); may be a partial loss of visual field
Dysarthria (slurred or indistinct speech)
Intense vertigo, double vision, unilateral hearing loss, nausea, vomiting, photophobia, or phonophobia

Reproduced with permission. CPR Issue, JAMA, October 28, 1992. © American Heart Association.

■ **Table 12.2**　**Assessment of the Patient with Acute Stroke**

Ensure adequate airway

　Measure vital signs frequently

　Conduct general medical assessment

　　Trauma of head or neck

　　Cardiovascular abnormalities

　　Ocular signs

　　Other signs

　Conduct neurologic examination

　　Level of consciousness

　　Glasgow Coma Scale (score 3–15)

　　Pupils

　　Individual limb movements

　　Meningeal signs

Reproduced with permission. CPR Issue, JAMA, October 28, 1992. © American Heart Asociation.

■ **Table 12.3**　**Initial Evaluation of a Patient with Acute Stroke**

CT of the brain without contrast

　ECG

　Chest roentgenogram

　Lateral cervical-spine roentgenogram (patients who are comatose or who have cervical spine pain or tenderness)

　Hematologic studies

　　Complete blood cell count

　　Platelet count

　　Prothrombin time

　　Partial thromboplastin time

　Serum electrolyte determinations (Na, K, Cl, bicarbonate)

　Blood glucose level

　Other chemical analyses

　Arterial blood gas levels

Reproduced with permission. CPR Issue, JAMA, October 28, 1992. © American Heart Association.

■ **Table 12.4**   **Emergency Treatment of a Stroke Patient**[a]

Contact neurologist or neurosurgeon

Fluid management (Class IIa)[b]
    Intravenous access
    Normal saline or lactated Ringer's at 30 mL/h
    Measure intake and output
    Slow infusion rate

Antihypertensive drugs: CT-guided therapy (Class IIa)
    Use rarely and cautiously in ischemic stroke
    Lower blood pressure to estimated prestroke levels in hemorrhagic stroke

Anticonvulsants (Class I)
    Phenytoin (15 mg/kg for adults) orally or IV; give no faster than 50 mg/
        min if administered IV
    Diazepam (10 mg IV for adults)
    Phenobarbital (15 mg/kg IV); use caution for respiratory depression

Treatment of increased intracranial pressure (Class I)
    Fluid restriction
    Intubation and hyperventilation to a PCO_2 of 25 to 28 mm Hg
    Mannitol support (1 to 2 g/kg IV over 5 to 10 min)
    Drainage of cerebrospinal fluid by intraventricular catheter
    Surgical intervention

Other interventions
    Surgery (Class 1)
    Clip aneurysm
    Resect arteriovenous malformation
    Evaluate hematoma
    Nimodipine for subarachnoid hemorrhage (Class I)

Anticoagulants (Class IIb)[c]

Thrombolytic drugs (Class IIb)[c]

New treatments for ischemic stroke[c]

[a] Class I, always acceptable, definitely effective; Class IIa, probably helpful; Class IIb, possibly helpful; Class III, possibly harmful, not indicated. Classes are defined fully on page 26.

[b] Class III if evidence of cerebral edema.

[c] Class III if evidence of hemorrhage.

Reproduced with permission. CPR Issue, JAMA, October 28, 1992. © American Heart Association.

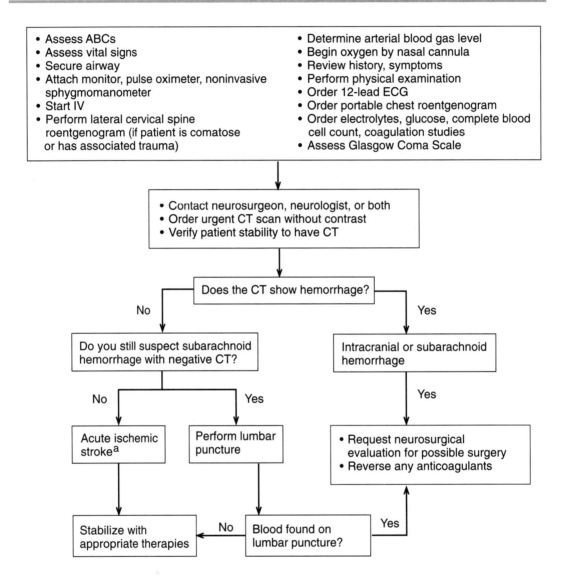

- Assess ABCs
- Assess vital signs
- Secure airway
- Attach monitor, pulse oximeter, noninvasive sphygmomanometer
- Start IV
- Perform lateral cervical spine roentgenogram (if patient is comatose or has associated trauma)

- Determine arterial blood gas level
- Begin oxygen by nasal cannula
- Review history, symptoms
- Perform physical examination
- Order 12-lead ECG
- Order portable chest roentgenogram
- Order electrolytes, glucose, complete blood cell count, coagulation studies
- Assess Glasgow Coma Scale

- Contact neurosurgeon, neurologist, or both
- Order urgent CT scan without contrast
- Verify patient stability to have CT

Does the CT show hemorrhage?

No · Yes

Do you still suspect subarachnoid hemorrhage with negative CT?

Intracranial or subarachnoid hemorrhage

No · Yes

Yes

Acute ischemic stroke[a]

Perform lumbar puncture

- Request neurosurgical evaluation for possible surgery
- Reverse any anticoagulants

Stabilize with appropriate therapies

No ← Blood found on lumbar puncture? → Yes

[a] The detailed management of acute stroke is beyond the scope of the ACLS program. Management of cardiovascular emergencies in stroke victims is similar to the management in other patients. Never forget, however, that acute stroke can coexist with acute cardiovascular problems.

■ **Figure 12.1**   Algorithm for initial evaluation of suspected stroke. Reproduced with permission. CPR Issue, JAMA, October 28, 1992. © American Heart Association.

Hypothermia

Severe accidental hypothermia continues to be an underappreciated cause of morbidity and mortality.[3] Victims may appear dead on initial evaluation due to marked depression of cardiovascular and brain function, but a full resuscitation with intact neurologic recovery is possible if appropriate measures are taken.[4] Clinical signs of death may be very misleading.

Key Points

- Never get into the cold water to assist a victim out of it—you will only end up with two victims! Use a ladder, stick, boat, rope, or other means to bring the victim to you.
- Loss of all pupil reflexes, absent BP, lack of respirations, hyporeflexia, and lack of any response to painful stimuli may *not* indicate clinical death in the hypothermic victim.
- Basic CPR should be initiated and continued in the pulseless patient with significant and profound bradycardia. The rate may need to be modified if extreme chest stiffness is present.
- All patients in cold-water rescues should have the following done:
  1. Remove wet garments and dry skin to prevent further core temperature loss.
  2. Prevent against heat loss and wind chill (insulate victims).
  3. Maintain horizontal position as much as possible to prevent aggravating potential orthostatic BP changes.
  4. Monitor cardiac rhythm.
  5. Monitor core temperature.
- Avoid all rough movements in the conscious, hypothermic victim as the cold heart is very susceptible to sudden jolts of activity and may end up in VF.
- For *conscious* victims being placed in a sleeping bag, pre-warm it by having a stripped-down volunteer crawl into it for several minutes. Cold sleeping bags will continue to draw core heat out of a hypothermic victim unless pre-warmed.

- Avoid all excessive movement or exercise in the *conscious*, hypothermic victim as this may cause peripheral vasodilation with shunting of cold blood from vasoconstricted limbs to the core (increasing *afterdrop*), potentially leading to an arrest situation (e.g., VF).
- Conscious hypothermic victims may be warmed with heat packs to the groin, neck, and armpits. **Never** use exercise in such victims for the reason stated above.
- Avoid giving hot fluids to conscious hypothermic victims in case unconsciousness later ensues as fluids in the stomach could then put them at risk for aspiration.
- In general, in the *unconscious* hypothermic victim whose core temperature is less than 31° C (88° F), all medications and invasive procedures (e.g., pacing wires, nasogastric tubes, etc.) should be avoided until core temperature is above 30° C (86°F).
- In unconscious hypothermic victims in VF whose core temperature is less than 31° C (88° F), it is not known at what temperature initial attempts at defibrillation should take place. A trial of 3 defibrillations (200 J, 300 J, 360 J) may be tried initially. If there is no response, *rewarming should be the treatment of choice* until the core temperatures rises to approximately 31° C (88° F).
- Always obtain *toxic screens on urine/blood* for all hypothermic victims as studies have shown a high proportion have ingested drugs (most commonly alcohol) and whose presence may complicate the resuscitation.
- Volume depletion is a common clinical finding in the severely hypothermic patient and warmed IV fluids are indicated. Due to significant peripheral vasoconstriction that exists in hypothermic victims, central line placement may be critical in order to infuse appropriate quantities of fluid.
- Conventional core rewarming techniques include the following:[3]
  1. Heated, humidified oxygen (warmed to 42° C to 46° C)
  2. Warmed IV fluids (normal saline) infused centrally at 43° C and at a rate of 150 to 200 mL/hr
  3. Peritoneal dialysis with warmed (43° C) potassium-free dialysate administered two liters at a time with no dwell time
  4. Extracorporeal rewarming (when/if available)
- Insulation of all warmed fluids (preferably normal saline) in liter bags and IV tubing is critical to prevent significant heat loss to the envi-

ronment (including room temperatures of 22° C (72° F). Wrap or insulate liter bags in insulating material (many commercial insulating bags are available) and place excess IV tubing under a blanket next to the victim's body if commercial IV line insulators are not used.

- If using microwave ovens to heat saline for infusion, always shake the bag before using, as microwaves heat from the inside out. It will take approximately 4 to 5 minutes on high power to heat one liter. Check the temperature of fluid before administering to see at what rate your particular oven heats the fluid. Hot tap water and conventional blood/fluid warmers may also be used.
- Extracorporeal rewarming is extremely useful for the rapid rewarming of hypothermic victims. Recently, arterial and venous catheters have been utilized to create a circulatory fistula through which blood can be heated by a commercially available countercurrent fluid warmer.[5]
- Although true hypothermic victims have a good chance of survival if resuscitative efforts are begun within 60 to 70 minutes, if there is pre-existing hypoxia prior to the victim becoming hypothermic (i.e., near-drowning episode), the likelihood for a good outcome is significantly diminished.
- **Never** use heating lamps, electric blankets, or hot packs to rewarm unconscious victims as this will cause peripheral vasodilation and shunt cold, lactic-acid–rich blood from the limbs *back* to the core and lower core temperature dramatically. This drop in core temperature may cause the death of the victim. Never use warm water enemas on *any* hypothermic as this may induce tremendous electrolyte imbalances. Gastric lavage is probably not effective as the surface area of the stomach is quite small compared to the large areas that can be covered with peritoneal lavage.
- Post-resuscitative complications include the following:[3]
  1. Pneumonia
  2. Pulmonary edema
  3. Acute tubular necrosis/renal failure
  4. Atrial arrhythmias
  5. Acute pancreatitis
  6. Disseminated intravascular coagulation
  7. Myoglobinuria
  8. Seizures

- Physicians must use their best clinical judgment to decide when resuscitative efforts should cease in a severely hypothermic arrest victim. Complete rewarming is *not* indicated in all victims, and chances for survival after 90 minutes of hypothermic cardiopulmonary arrest are extremely low.

Summary

The introduction of a new AHA algorithm for the treatment of severe hypothermia will help teach the basic assessment and rewarming techniques required by emergency providers. Although there is limited field ability to accomplish definitive rewarming, stabilization prior to transport to an appropriate facility is possible. Close post-resuscitative management is required for all hypothermic victims as respiratory and other organ system complications may occur.

Figure 12.2 shows the algorithm for treatment of hypothemia.

Near-Drowning

Key Points

The end stage of all drowning episodes is hypoxia with subsequent brain damage and death. The duration of the hypoxia is the key factor in determining outcome.

- Rescue breathing should be initiated on all near-drowning victims.
- If a diving accident is suspected, always assume a neck injury exists until proven otherwise. Support the victim's neck in a neutral position (without flexion or extension) and the victim should be floated supine on a back board prior to removal from the water. Use jaw thrust without head tilt for rescue breathing.
- There is no need to clear the airway of aspirated water. However, you may need to remove gastric contents, foreign materials, or other debris using standard techniques for an obstructed airway. Some people be-

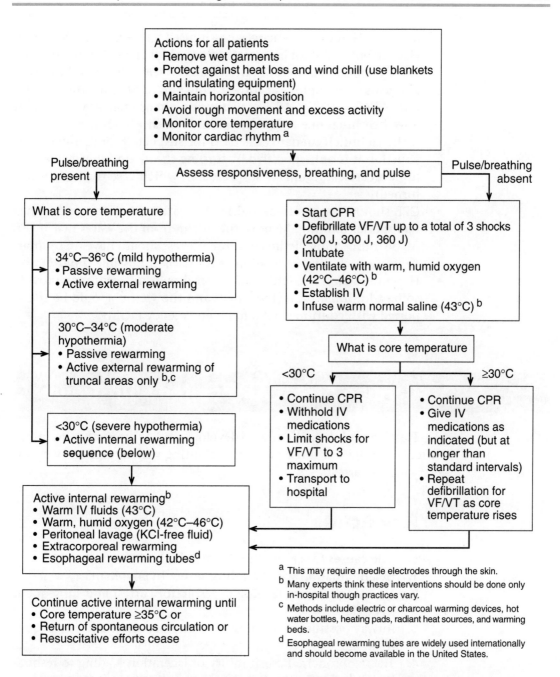

Figure 12.2   Algorithm for treatment of hypothermia. Reproduced with permission. CPR Issue, JAMA, October 28, 1992. © American Heart Association.

lieve the Heimlich maneuver has limited value in near-drowning victims, but it has not been recommended for all victims by the AHA as only a modest amount of fresh water or sea water is in the airway and usually is rapidly absorbed from the lungs into the circulation.[1,6,7] Also, 10% to 12% of victims do not aspirate any fluid at all into their lungs due to laryngospasm or breath-holding.[6,7]

- If the Heimlich maneuver is used for suspected foreign-body obstruction it is only modified by turning the victim's head sideways (unless cervical trauma is suspected, in which case the head is not turned).
- CPR should *not* be attempted in the water unless the rescuer has had special training. Remove the victim from the water first.
- All near-drowning victims in cardiac arrest should have ACLS interventions including intubation at the earliest possible time.
- Hypothermia in the setting of a near-drowning event may provide some additional protective effect and the victim should be transported with continued CPR to an emergency facility.

Cardiac Arrest Associated with Trauma

Treatment of the patient who develops cardiac arrest after an injury differs from that for those patients presenting with a respiratory or primary cardiac arrest.

Key Points

- Possible causes for cardiac arrest include the following:
  1. Exsanguination with resulting severe hypovolemia
  2. Neurologic injury leading to respiratory arrest and subsequent hypoxia
  3. Airway obstruction leading to respiratory arrest and subsequent hypoxia
  4. Tracheobronchial crush injury or laceration leading to respiratory arrest and subsequent hypoxia
  5. Severe, direct injuries to the aorta or heart

6. Cardiovascular collapse secondary to severe central neurologic injury
7. Tension pneumothorax or pericardial tamponade leading to reduced cardiac output
8. Injuries accompanied by severe hypothermia

- Outcome may be quite guarded depending on the severity of the illness, although some problems (tamponade, tension pneumothorax) may be reversed fairly easily.
- Attempt to resuscitate a patient with a primary cardiac arrhythmia whose injury is secondary.
- Direct initial efforts at potentially reversible conditions that are affecting ventilation, cardiac output or oxygenation.
- Arrange immediate transport of all patients for definitive evaluation and therapy.
- Hypothermic patients may have ability to sustain extended periods of pulselessness and need definitive evaluation and rewarming as indicated.
- Do not attempt resuscitation in patients with decapitation, patients with severe blunt trauma without any vital signs, or victims exhibiting no pupillary responses (except in hypothermic victims).
- In patients undergoing resuscitation, airway assessment and ventilation should *always* be an ongoing priority! Intubate if possible!
- Always rule out an occult neck injury prior to movement of the neck.
- Chest compressions, airway control, and defibrillation should be utilized in appropriate clinical situations in patients presenting with trauma-associated cardiac arrest.

Electric Shock and Lightning

Approximately 500 to 1,000 deaths per year occur due to electric shocks and about 50 to 300 fatalities due to lightning strikes. The spectrum of injuries can vary from minimal damage to cardiac arrest. The magnitude and duration of current correlate best with the extent of injury. Due to the fact that current can travel along blood vessels and nerves easily, extensive damage to underlying tissues may result and a burn/surgical specialist should be consulted at the earliest possible time in electrical injuries. Remember, the superficial skin of the victim may appear relatively untouched initially and only in the subsequent 24 to 48 hours will massive underlying skin necrosis appear.

Key Points

- Alternating current can cause VF due to the likelihood of current exposure during the recovery period of the cardiac cycle.
- Cardiopulmonary arrest is the primary cause of immediate death.
- Vigorous resuscitative measures are indicated for victims of electric shock.
- *Always* turn off electrical source, avoid contact with exposed wires.
- Cardiopulmonary resuscitation is initiated on all victims not breathing.
- Secure the airway and provide supplemental oxygen.
- Follow all ACLS algorithms for arrhythmias determined on evaluation of victim.
- Rapid IV infusions of saline are indicated for victims with hypovolemic shock and to maintain a diuresis to help avoid renal shutdown secondary to myoglobinuria.
- In lightning-strike victims, cardiac arrest is due to either VF or asystole, although sometimes organized cardiac activity may return spontaneously.
- Rescuers should give highest priority when there are multiple lightning strike victims to those in respiratory or cardiac arrest, as victims who initially survive a strike will rarely later suffer a cardiac arrest.

Pregnancy

Pregnancy renders the woman more susceptible to major cardiovascular and respiratory insults. Events that may cause cardiac arrest in pregnancy include trauma, pulmonary embolism, cardiac disease, peripartum hemorrhage with secondary hypovolemia, and amniotic fluid embolism.

When cardiac arrest occurs during pregnancy, all standard CPR and ACLS guidelines should be followed *without* modification. If there is reason to believe there is fetal viability, rapid performance of a perimortem cesarean section should be considered if CPR and ACLS interventions have failed to restore effective circulation. Obstetric and neonatal personnel should be called immediately.

References

1. American Heart Association. Guidelines for cardiopulmonary resuscitation and emergency cardiac care. *JAMA* 1992;268:2171–2302.
2. Teasdale G, Jennett B. Assessment of coma and impaired consciousness: A practical scale. *Lancet* 1974;2:81–84.
3. Weinberg AD. Hypothermia. *Ann Emerg Med* 1993;22 (pt 2):370–377.
4. Fox RH, Woodward PM, Exton-Smith AN, et al. Body temperature in the elderly: A national study of physiological, social and environmental conditions. *Br Med J* 1973;1:200–206.
5. Gentilello LM, Rifley WJ. Continuous arteriovenous rewarming: Report of a new technique for treating hypothermia. *J Trauma* 1991;31:1151–1154.
6. Modell JH, Davis JH. Electrolyte changes in human drowning victims. *Anesthesiology* 1969;30:414–420.
7. Modell, JH. Is the Heimlich maneuver appropriate as first treatment for drowning? *Emerg Med Serv* 1981;10:63–66.

Notes

13 Let's Put It All Together

Objectives

1. Determine the role and responsibilities of the code team leader.
2. Summarize the new algorithms developed by the AHA for use in cardiopulmonary arrests:
   - Ventricular fibrillation and pulseless VT
   - Asystole
   - Pulseless electrical activity/EMD
   - Ventricular tachycardia
   - Paroxysmal supraventricular tachycardia
   - Atrial fibrillation/atrial flutter
3. Explain the recommended approach to post-resuscitation care.
4. Identify some of the difficulties health-care professionals face when conveying the news of a death to a family member.
5. Describe the AHA recommendations concerning Critical Incident Debriefing.

Overview

Putting all the information one has learned during an ACLS course together can be difficult. The integration of knowledge, psychomotor skills, and common sense can stress even the coolest of heads. This chapter will attempt to summarize the major principles of conducting a successful code and will review again some of the specific treatment algorithms of ACLS. A good team leader is an excellent organizer and supervisor and must assimilate data in the midst of "organized chaos" at times.

Not everyone can be an outstanding leader, but, by practicing being a team leader during an ACLS course, much of the anxiety can be diminished. A team leader in control can many times also calm the anxieties of the other members of the team. Even though you may never actually be a team leader, it is critical to experience the stress and difficulties of having this position.

Responsibilities of the Code Team Leader

- Supervises all aspects of the team's actions
- Monitors ventilation and intubation attempts
- Evaluates adequacy of CPR efforts
- Directs appropriate AHA algorithm
- Orders appropriate medications in the correct dose
- Ensures safety of all team members
- Orders and interprets laboratory data, including cardiac rhythm
- Evaluates any equipment malfunctioning
- Ensures good crowd control and effects overall leadership of patient care
- Communicates his or her observations, diagnoses, and planned interventions and encourages suggestions from team members

Key Points

- Always check equipment, especially defibrillator equipment, prior to assuming code responsibilities.
- Make sure you know who your code team members are *before* a code is called!

- Always check beepers and paging information to ensure open communication in case of emergency.
- Always allow time after a code to review the team's performance and allow feedback and educational items to be discussed.
- ***Do not*** interrupt CPR for longer than 15 s to 30 s, even for placement of lines or tubes or for transport of a patient.
- Any tachycardic rhythm that is producing hemodynamic instability should be countershocked as soon as a defibrillator is available. The more unstable the dysrhythmia, the more urgent is the necessity for the shock.
- There are three main reasons a patient's BP can be low: (1) a rate problem, (2) a pump problem, or (3) a volume problem. In general, try to correct the *rate* first before treating any pump or volume problems (e.g., if a patient is hypotensive and bradycardic, try to increase the heart rate before using any inotropes, pressors, or fluids). In general, if the lungs are clear it is usually preferable to give fluids before using any pressor agents.
- For patients in VF, treatment of choice is defibrillation (see below under "Comments" section for VF/pulseless VT algorithm).
- For patients experiencing extreme clinical conditions or in pulseless VT, an *unsynchronized* countershock may be administered. When the patient has an AV block or bradycardia, the first priority is to correct any underlying causes (i.e., hypoxia, electrolyte disturbances). Correction of known abnormalities should precede reliance on atropine or even pacing. Catecholamines should only be used until a pacemaker can be inserted as soon as practicable.
- ***Do not*** use lidocaine or bretylium to suppress ventricular escape rhythms. The correct treatment for any underlying and significant bradycardia with ventricular ectopy is either atropine (to increase heart rate) or immediate pacing. Suppression of ventricular escape beats with antiarrhythmics may totally extinguish ventricular activity.
- For significant bradycardias or high-level AV blocks, rapid order of external pacing by the team leader is indicated. External pacing may have some role also in those patients with asystole, although the best response is obtained only in those with a short duration of being in asystole.

- When ordering epinephrine for administration through an ET tube, note that a dose of at least 2 to 2.5 times the peripheral IV dose may be required.
- The ordering of high-dose epinephrine (used in studies with doses of between 0.1 and 0.2 mg/kg, which is 10 to 20 times the usual dose of epinephrine) has *not* been endorsed by the AHA and its use is neither encouraged nor discouraged for those patients failing to respond to standard doses. Note that these recommendations pertain to adults only and not to children. Pediatric epinephrine administration (first dose) is still 0.01 mg/kg while the second dose has been increased to 0.1 to 0.2 mg/kg and is administered 3 to 5 minutes after the initial dose.
- When ordering atropine, remember it will most likely be effective when the block is at the AV node or higher or when there is a definite vagal component causing the bradydysrhythmia. Some patients may need a total of 3.0 mg ordered (recommended in asystole) by the team leader to achieve a full vagolytic dose.
- **Do not** order adenosine for atrial fibrillation! It is not indicated for either this arrhythmia or atrial flutter. Adenosine is considered the drug of choice for narrow-complex PSVT.
- **Do not** order verapamil for wide-complex tachycardias or WPW syndrome. Verapamil can be used to break PSVT, but it will only slow the ventricular response for atrial fibrillation and atrial flutter.

Review of Key AHA Algorithms

This section will cover the key AHA algorithms with commentary that is critical to overall management of a majority of emergency resuscitations.

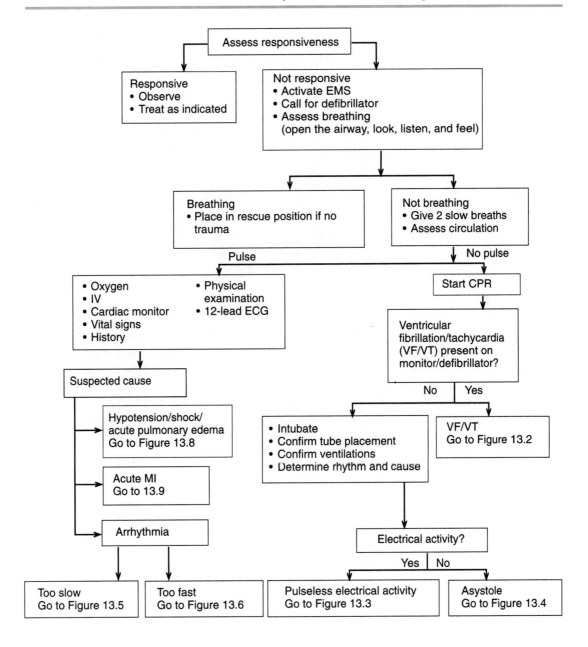

■ **Figure 13.1**   Universal algorithm for adult emergency cardiac care (ECC). Reproduced with permission. CPR Issue, JAMA, October 28, 1992. © American Heart Association.

Comments on Algorithm

1. All resuscitation efforts should *always* start with this algorithm.
2. Always activate the EMS system when you find the patient unresponsive outside of a hospital setting and the code team when you are in a hospital.
3. If a flat line appears on the monitor, check for
   - Loose leads
   - Improper connection to the patient
   - No patient connection to the defibrillator or monitor
   - Power not turned on
   - Isoelectric VF/VT
   - Asystole present
4. Always check your defibrillator machine (at least daily) to ensure proper functioning *before* you have to use it. Operator errors and poor equipment maintenance account for the vast majority of defibrillator failures.

■ **Figure 13.2**   Algorithm for ventricular fibrillation and pulseless ventricular tachycardia (VF/VT). Reproduced with permission. CPR Issue, JAMA, October 28, 1992. © American Heart Association.

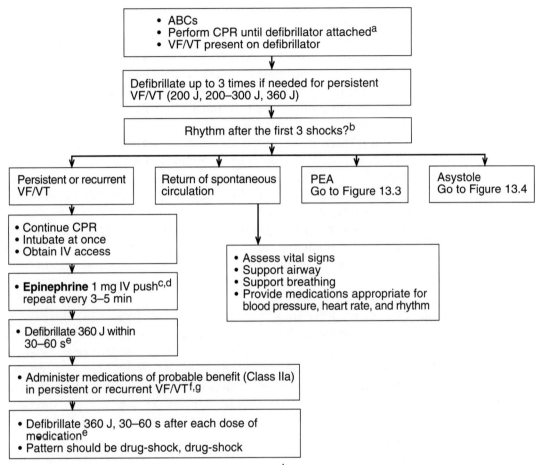

- ABCs
- Perform CPR until defibrillator attached[a]
- VF/VT present on defibrillator

Defibrillate up to 3 times if needed for persistent VF/VT (200 J, 200–300 J, 360 J)

Rhythm after the first 3 shocks?[b]

| Persistent or recurrent VF/VT | Return of spontaneous circulation | PEA Go to Figure 13.3 | Asystole Go to Figure 13.4 |

Persistent or recurrent VF/VT:
- Continue CPR
- Intubate at once
- Obtain IV access

- **Epinephrine** 1 mg IV push[c,d] repeat every 3–5 min

- Defibrillate 360 J within 30–60 s[e]

- Administer medications of probable benefit (Class IIa) in persistent or recurrent VF/VT[f,g]

- Defibrillate 360 J, 30–60 s after each dose of medication[e]
- Pattern should be drug-shock, drug-shock

Return of spontaneous circulation:
- Assess vital signs
- Support airway
- Support breathing
- Provide medications appropriate for blood pressure, heart rate, and rhythm

Class I: definitely helpful

Class IIa: acceptable, probably helpful

Class IIb: acceptable, possibly helpful

Class III: not indicated, may be harmful

[a] Precordial thump is a Class IIb action in witnessed arrest, no pulse, and no defibrillator immediately available.

[b] Hypothermic cardiac arrest is treated differently after this point. See section on hypothermia.

[c] The recommended dose of **epinephrine** is 1 mg IV push every 3–5 min. If this approach fails, several Class IIb dosing regimens can be considered
- Intermediate: **epinephrine** 2–5 mg IV push every 3–5 min
- Escalating: **epinephrine** 1 mg–3 mg–5 mg IV push (3 min apart)
- High: **epinephrine** 0.1 mg/kg IV push, every 3–5 min

[d] **Sodium bicarbonate** (1 mEq/kg) is Class I if patient has known preexisting hyperkalemia

[e] Multiple sequenced shocks (200 J, 200–300 J, 360 J) are acceptable here (Class I), especially when medications are delayed

[f]
- **Lidocaine** 1.5 mg/kg IV push. Repeat in 3–5 min to total loading dose of 3 mg/kg then use
- **Bretylium** 5 mg/kg IV push. Repeat in 5 min at 10 mg/kg
- **Magnesium sulfate** 1–2 g IV in torsades de pointes or suspected hypomagnesemic state or severe refractory VF
- **Procainamide** 30 mg/min in refractory VF (maximum total 17 mg/kg)

[g]
- **Sodium bicarbonate** (1 mEq/kg IV):
  Class IIa
  - if known preexisting bicarbonate-responsive acidosis
  - if overdose with tricyclic antidepressants
  - to alkalinize the urine in drug overdoses
  Class IIb
  - if intubated and continued long arrest interval
  - upon return of spontaneous circulation after long arrest interval
  Class III
  - hypoxic lactic acidosis

Comments on Algorithm

1. For persistent VF and pulseless VT, defibrillate up to three times consecutively, and CPR should *not* be performed between delivery of these shocks. Successful resuscitation from VF depends on aggressive initial efforts. Defibrillation for VF may *precede* airway, breathing, and circulation in many clinical circumstances. Automatic external defibrillators may play an increasingly important role in resuscitation provided by first responders in the field and you should understand the uses and limitations of AEDs (see Chapter 9, Electrical Therapy and How to Use It).

2. Do *not* pause for a pulse check if a properly connected monitor clearly shows persistent VF/VT.

3. Always remove nitroglycerin patches (if time permits) to prevent possible electrical arcing.

4. Always avoid placing defibrillator paddles over the generator unit of implanted pacemakers (should be approximately 5 inches from generator packs).

5. The team leader should always announce in a loud, clear voice when defibrillation is going to be accomplished so team members can clear themselves of any contact with the patient or the bed.

6. Epinephrine in a dose of 1 mg IV every 3 to 5 minutes continues to be the first line agent recommended. Repeat doses early if clinical response is unsatisfactory. A higher dose (5 mg, or approximately 0.1 mg/kg) should *only* be used if the lower dose has failed to produce the desired clinical results.

7. During cardiac arrest, if lidocaine is ordered only bolus therapy should be used until return of spontaneous circulation. After restoration of circulation, a continuous infusion at 2 to 4 mg/min can then be started.

8. Human clinical studies have not shown either lidocaine or bretylium to be superior over the other.

9. Sodium bicarbonate continues to be recommended *only* when the clinical situation indicates its need as determined by arterial blood gas analysis.

10. Known or suspected hyperkalemia (serum potassium levels >6 mmol/L) should be treated with calcium chloride 4 mg/kg IV.

PEA includes	• Electromechanical dissociation (EMD)
	• Pseudo-EMD
	• Idioventricular rhythms
	• Ventricular escape rhythms
	• Bradyasystolic rhythms
	• Postdefibrillation idioventricular rhythms

• Continue CPR
• Intubate at once
• Obtain IV access
• Assess blood flow using Doppler ultrasound

↓

Consider possible causes (Parentheses = possible therapies and treatments)
• Hypovolemia (volume infusion)
• Hypoxia (ventilation)
• Cardiac tamponade (pericardiocentesis)
• Tension pneumothorax (needle decompression)
• Hypothermia (see Chapter 12)
• Massive pulmonary embolism (surgery, **thrombolytics**)
• Drug overdoses such as tricyclics, digitalis, ß-blockers, calcium channel blockers
• Hyperkalemia [a]
• Acidosis [b]
• Massive acute myocardial infarction (go to Figure 13.9)

↓

• **Epinephrine** 1 mg IV push,[a,c] repeat every 3–5 min

↓

• If absolute bradycardia (<60 beats/min) or relative bradycardia, give **atropine** 1 mg IV
• Repeat every 3–5 min up to a total of 0.04 mg/kg[d]

Class I: definitely helpful
Class IIa: acceptable, probably helpful
Class IIb: acceptable, possibly helpful
Class III: not indicated, may be harmful
[a] **Sodium bicarbonate** 1 mEq/kg is Class I if patient has known preexisting hyperkalemia.
[b] **Sodium bicarbonate** 1 mEq/kg:
Class IIa
• if known preexisting bicarbonate-responsive acidosis
• if overdose with tricyclic antidepressants
• to alkalinize the urine in drug overdoses
Class IIb
• if intubated and long arrest interval
• upon return of spontaneous circulation after long arrest interval

Class III
• hypoxic lactic acidosis
[c] The recommended dose of **epinephrine** is 1 mg IV push every 3–5 min. If this approach fails, several Class IIb dosing regimens can be considered.
• Intermediate: **epinephrine** 2–5 mg IV push every 3–5 min
• Escalating: **epinephrine** 1 mg-3 mg-5 mg IV push (3 min apart)
• High: **epinephrine** 0.1 mg/kg IV push every 3–5 min
[d] Shorter **atropine** dosing intervals are possibly helpful in cardiac arrest (Class IIb).

■ **Figure 13.3** **Algorithm for pulseless electrical activity (PEA) (electromechanical dissociation [EMD]). Reproduced with permission. CPR Issue, JAMA, October 28, 1992. © American Heart Association.**

Comments on Algorithm

1. The term *pulseless electrical activity* includes EMD and a group of rhythms including the following:
   - Pseudo-EMD (see below)
   - Idioventricular rhythms
   - Ventricular escape rhythms
   - Post-defibrillation idioventricular rhythms
   - Bradyasystolic rhythms
2. Pseudo-EMD is the new term associated with the finding that electrical activity often is associated with mechanical contractions that are too weak to produce a detectable BP, which differs from the traditional view that there is a lack of myocardial muscle fiber shortening.
3. A summary of causes of PEA, many of which are reversible, include the following:
   - Hypovolemia (most common)
   - Cardiac tamponade
   - Tension pneumothorax
   - Massive pulmonary embolism
   - Hypoventilation/hypoxemia
   - Acidosis/electrolyte imbalances (severe hyperkalemia)
   - Hypothermia
   - Many different drug overdoses
4. Patients with Doppler-detectable blood flow should be treated with the algorithm for severe hypotension (BP < 70 mm Hg).
5. Fluid challenges can be used to treat suspected hypovolemia.
6. Finding the underlying etiology and instituting appropriate treatment for PEA is the only definitive method to treat the patient!

■ **Figure 13.4**   Asystole treatment algorithm. Reproduced with permission. CPR Issue, ▶
JAMA, October 28, 1992. © American Heart Association.

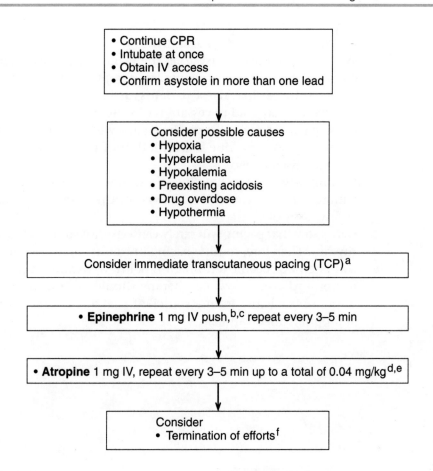

• Continue CPR
• Intubate at once
• Obtain IV access
• Confirm asystole in more than one lead

Consider possible causes
• Hypoxia
• Hyperkalemia
• Hypokalemia
• Preexisting acidosis
• Drug overdose
• Hypothermia

Consider immediate transcutaneous pacing (TCP)[a]

• **Epinephrine** 1 mg IV push,[b,c] repeat every 3–5 min

• **Atropine** 1 mg IV, repeat every 3–5 min up to a total of 0.04 mg/kg[d,e]

Consider
• Termination of efforts[f]

Class I: definitely helpful

Class IIa: acceptable, probably helpful

Class IIb: acceptable, possibly helpful

Class III: not indicated, may be harmful

[a] TCP is a Class IIb intervention. Lack of success may be due to delays in pacing. To be effective TCP must be performed early, simultaneously with drugs. Evidence does not support routine use of TCP for asystole.

[b] The recommended dose of **epinephrine** is 1 mg IV push every 3–5 min. If this approach fails, several Class IIb dosing regimens can be considered:
 • Intermediate: **epinephrine** 2–5 mg IV push every 3–5 min
 • Escalating: **epinephrine** 1 mg-3 mg-5 mg IV push (3 min apart)
 • High: **epinephrine** 0.1 mg/kg IV push every 3–5 min

[c] **Sodium bicarbonate** 1 mEq/kg is Class I if patient has known preexisting hyperkalemia.

[d] Shorter **atropine** dosing intervals are Class IIb in asystolic arrest.

[e] **Sodium bicarbonate** 1 mEq/kg
Class IIa
 • if known preexisting bicarbonate-responsive acidosis
 • if overdose with tricyclic antidepressants
 • to alkalinize the urine in drug overdoses
Class IIb
 • if intubated and continued long arrest interval
 • upon return of spontaneous circulation after long arrest interval
Class III
 • hypoxic lactic acidosis

[f] If patient remains in asystole or other agonal rhythms after successful intubation and initial medications and no reversible causes are identified, consider termination of resuscitative efforts by a physician. Consider interval since arrest.

Comments on Algorithm

1. With the diagnosis of asystole, the team leader must aggressively consider the differential diagnosis. Atropine is routinely given to all asystolic cardiac arrest patients, as high levels of parasympathetic tone may lead to cessation of ventricular activity.

2. Electric shocks may also produce parasympathetic discharge and, for this reason, routine defibrillation of true asystole should be strongly discouraged.

3. Confirm asystole by changing to a second lead. Operator errors are a more common cause of false asystole than are fine VF appearing as false asystole.

4. Data show that pacing will rarely cause asystole to revert to a normal rhythm. Therefore, routine pacing in true asystole is *not* justified.

5. Although no specific termination point for treatment can be given in normothermic asystole, therapy should be continued until no response is elicited from a sufficient trial of CPR, intubation, and appropriate medications.

■ **Figure 13.5** Bradycardia algorithm (with the patient not in cardiac arrest). Reproduced with permission. CPR Issue, JAMA, October 28, 1992. © American Heart Association. ▶

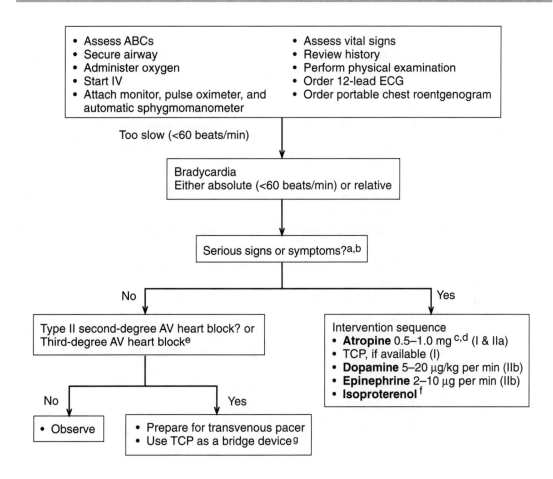

- Assess ABCs
- Secure airway
- Administer oxygen
- Start IV
- Attach monitor, pulse oximeter, and automatic sphygmomanometer

- Assess vital signs
- Review history
- Perform physical examination
- Order 12-lead ECG
- Order portable chest roentgenogram

Too slow (<60 beats/min)

Bradycardia
Either absolute (<60 beats/min) or relative

Serious signs or symptoms?[a,b]

No

Type II second-degree AV heart block? or Third-degree AV heart block[e]

No

- Observe

Yes

- Prepare for transvenous pacer
- Use TCP as a bridge device[g]

Yes

Intervention sequence
- **Atropine** 0.5–1.0 mg [c,d] (I & IIa)
- TCP, if available (I)
- **Dopamine** 5–20 µg/kg per min (IIb)
- **Epinephrine** 2–10 µg per min (IIb)
- **Isoproterenol** [f]

[a] Serious signs or symptoms must be related to the slow rate. Clinical manifestations include *symptoms* (chest pain, shortness of breath, decreased level of consciousness) and *signs* (low BP, shock, pulmonary congestion, CHF, acute MI).

[b] Do not delay TCP while awaiting IV access or for **atropine** to take effect if patient is symptomatic.

[c] Denervated transplanted hearts will not respond to **atropine**. Go at once to pacing, **catecholamine** infusion, or both.

[d] **Atropine** should be given in repeat doses in 3–5 min up to total of 0.04 mg/kg. Consider shorter dosing intervals in severe clinical conditions. It

has been suggested that atropine should be used with caution in atrioventricular (AV) block at the His-Purkinje level (type II AV block and new third-degree block with wide QRS complexes) (Class IIb).

[e] Never treat third-degree heart block plus ventricular escape beats with **lidocaine**.

[f] **Isoproterenol** should be used, if at all, with extreme caution. At low doses it is Class IIb (possibly helpful); at higher doses it is Class III (harmful).

[g] Verify patient tolerance and mechanical capture. Use analgesia and sedation as needed.

Comments on Algorithm

1. It is important when evaluating a patient with bradycardia to assess the patient and not treat the monitor. The term *relative bradycardia* refers to the situation where the BP is too low relative to the heart rate (HR). If the low HR is making the patient ill, treatment is indicated. Clinical manifestations of bradycardia include
    *   Chest pain
    *   Shortness of breath
    *   Decreased level of consciousness
    *   Hypotension
    *   Congestive heart failure
    *   Premature ventricular contractions (PVCs) in the setting of an acute MI

2. Lidocaine used on ventricular escape beats misdiagnosed as PVCs or slow VT may be **lethal**.

3. Hypotension associated with bradycardia (if due to hypovolemia or myocardial dysfunction) should not be treated by artificially attempting to increase the HR.

4. In addition to transcutaneous pacing, an epinephrine infusion can be started for patients with severe bradycardia associated with hypotension (see Table 11.1, ACLS Drug Chart, for concentration and dose).

5. Isoproterenol continues to be **not** recommended for patients with severe symptomatic bradycardia. Isoproterenol produces negative effects of increased myocardial oxygen consumption.

6. Patients with third-degree AV block in conjunction with anterior-wall infarct should have a transvenous pacemaker inserted. Symptomatic patients should be initially treated with transcutaneous pacing, dopamine, and epinephrine. Atropine is **contraindicated**.

■ **Figure 13.6** Tachycardia algorithm. Reproduced with permission. CPR Issue, JAMA, ▶ October 28, 1992. © American Heart Association.

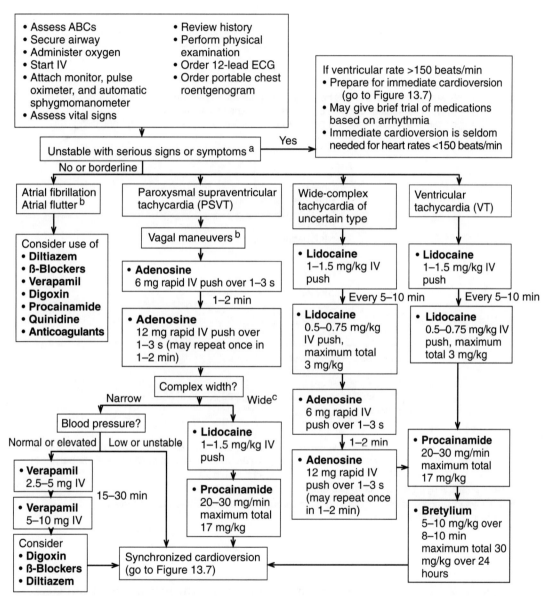

a Unstable condition must be related to the tachycardia. Signs and symptoms may include chest pain, shortness of breath, decreased level of consciousness, low blood pressure (BP), shock, pulmonary congestion, congestive heart failure, acute myocardial infarction.

b Carotid sinus pressure is contraindicated in patients with carotid bruits, avoid ice-water immersion in patients with ischemic heart disease.

c If the wide-complex tachycardia is known with certainty to be PSVT and BP is normal/elevated, sequence can include **verapamil**.

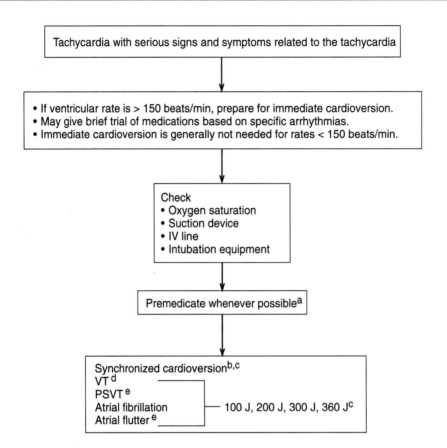

Tachycardia with serious signs and symptoms related to the tachycardia

- If ventricular rate is > 150 beats/min, prepare for immediate cardioversion.
- May give brief trial of medications based on specific arrhythmias.
- Immediate cardioversion is generally not needed for rates < 150 beats/min.

Check
- Oxygen saturation
- Suction device
- IV line
- Intubation equipment

Premedicate whenever possible[a]

Synchronized cardioversion[b,c]
VT [d]
PSVT [e]
Atrial fibrillation
Atrial flutter [e] ——— 100 J, 200 J, 300 J, 360 J[c]

[a] Effective regimens have included a sedative (e.g., **diazepam, midazolam, barbiturates, etomidate, ketamine, methohexital**) with or without an analgesic agent (e.g., **fentanyl, morphine, meperidine**). Many experts recommend anesthesia if service is readily available.

[b] Note possible need to resynchronize after each cardioversion.

[c] If delays in synchronization occur and clinical conditions are critical, go to immediate unsynchronized shocks.

[d] Treat polymorphic VT (irregular form and rate) like VF: 200 J, 200–300 J, 360 J.

[e] PSVT and atrial flutter often respond to lower energy levels (start with 50 J).

Figure 13.7 Electrical cardioversion algorithm (with the patient not in cardiac arrest). Reproduced with permission. CPR Issue, JAMA, October 28, 1992. © American Heart Association.

Comments on Algorithms

1. Clinicians must differentiate whether it is the tachycardia itself producing the patient's symptoms or the underlying disease/illness causing the tachycardia. Adverse clinical hemodynamic symptoms seen in patients with tachycardia include
   * Hypotension
   * Symptoms of CHF
   * Decreased level of consciousness
   * Persistent chest pain
   * Continued PVCs in setting of acute MI

2. Cardioversion remains the primary treatment for the hemodynamically unstable patient with tachycardia and precedes antiarrhythmic therapy. All patients for cardioversion should be attached to a monitor and an oxygen source, and have an IV line in place.

3. New-onset atrial fibrillation can indicate a silent ischemic event or hyperthyroidism in the elderly.

4. Patients with atrial fibrillation for more than a few days may develop intra-atrial thrombi and should receive anticoagulation therapy before any pharmacologic or electrical conversion interventions.

5. Adenosine is as effective as verapamil in initial conversion of PSVT and produces less hypotension. Because of its short half-life, it is considered the safer agent.

6. Hypotension secondary to verapamil use can be reversed with calcium chloride 0.5 to 1.0 gm IV given slowly. Routine pretreatment of patients with calcium prior to treatment with verapamil is *not* recommended due to insufficient data.

7. Administration of verapamil to a patient with VT can be **lethal.** It can accelerate heart rate and decrease blood pressure. Verapamil should also not be given to patients with a wide-complex tachycardia unless it is due to a supraventricular origin without question. Verapamil should always be used with caution in patients receiving IV or chronic beta-blocker medication.

8. Synchronized cardioversion should be accomplished when the patient is stable and has a tachycardia with a rate < 160 beats per minute. Defibrillation (*unsynchronized* shock) would be indicated in a patient considered clinically unstable with a rapid tachycardia and when delays in synchronized cardioversion occur (see Figure 13.7).

9. **Always** consider sedation for any patient on whom you will be performing elective or urgent cardioversion. If anesthesia personnel cannot be present, consider the use of IV diazepam. The procedure is not painless and patients not sedated will often have a vivid and unpleasant memory of the event.

■ **Figure 13.8**   Algorithm for hypotension, shock, and acute pulmonary edema. Repro- ▶ duced with permission. CPR Issue, JAMA, October 28, 1992. © American Heart Association.

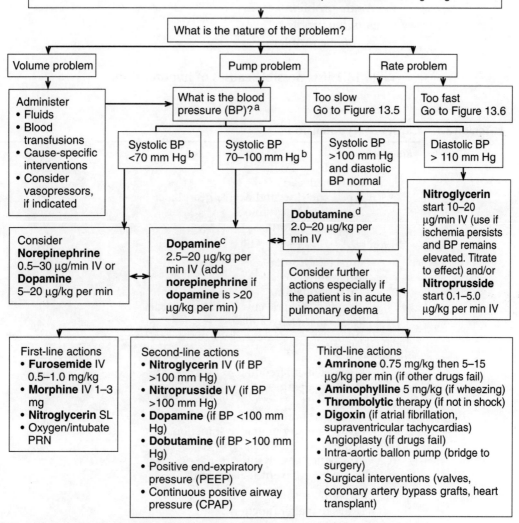

Clinical signs of hypoperfusion, congestive heart failure, acute pulmonary edema
- Assess ABCs
- Secure airway
- Administer oxygen
- Start IV

- Attach monitor, pulse oximeter, automatic sphygmomanometer
- Assess vital signs
- Review history
- Perform physical examination
- Order 12-lead ECG
- Order portable chest roentgenogram

What is the nature of the problem?

Volume problem | **Pump problem** | **Rate problem**

Administer
- Fluids
- Blood transfusions
- Cause-specific interventions
- Consider vasopressors, if indicated

What is the blood pressure (BP)?[a]

Too slow
Go to Figure 13.5

Too fast
Go to Figure 13.6

Systolic BP <70 mm Hg[b]

Systolic BP 70–100 mm Hg[b]

Systolic BP >100 mm Hg and diastolic BP normal

Diastolic BP > 110 mm Hg

Nitroglycerin start 10–20 µg/min IV (use if ischemia persists and BP remains elevated. Titrate to effect) and/or **Nitroprusside** start 0.1–5.0 µg/kg per min IV

Dobutamine[d] 2.0–20 µg/kg per min IV

Consider **Norepinephrine** 0.5–30 µg/min IV or **Dopamine** 5–20 µg/kg per min

Dopamine[c] 2.5–20 µg/kg per min IV (add **norepinephrine** if **dopamine** is >20 µg/kg per min)

Consider further actions especially if the patient is in acute pulmonary edema

First-line actions
- **Furosemide** IV 0.5–1.0 mg/kg
- **Morphine** IV 1–3 mg
- **Nitroglycerin** SL
- Oxygen/intubate PRN

Second-line actions
- **Nitroglycerin** IV (if BP >100 mm Hg)
- **Nitroprusside** IV (if BP >100 mm Hg)
- **Dopamine** (if BP <100 mm Hg)
- **Dobutamine** (if BP >100 mm Hg)
- Positive end-expiratory pressure (PEEP)
- Continuous positive airway pressure (CPAP)

Third-line actions
- **Amrinone** 0.75 mg/kg then 5–15 µg/kg per min (if other drugs fail)
- **Aminophylline** 5 mg/kg (if wheezing)
- **Thrombolytic** therapy (if not in shock)
- **Digoxin** (if atrial fibrillation, supraventricular tachycardias)
- Angioplasty (if drugs fail)
- Intra-aortic ballon pump (bridge to surgery)
- Surgical interventions (valves, coronary artery bypass grafts, heart transplant)

[a] Base management after this point on invasive hemodynamic monitoring if possible.
[b] Fluid bolus of 250–500 mL normal saline should be tried. If no response, consider sympathomimetics.
[c] Move to **dopamine** and stop **norepinephrine** when BP improves.
[d] Add **dopamine** when BP improves. Avoid **dobutamine** when systolic BP <100 mm Hg.

Comments on Algorithm

1. Shock is a syndrome where there is inadequate oxygen delivery and cellular perfusion for existing metabolic demands. Determining and correcting the underlying etiology for the shock syndrome is critical.
2. The causes of hypotension can be simplified as follows:
   * A *rate* problem
   * A *pump* problem
   * A *volume* problem

   Table 13.1 lists possible causes of hypotension.

■ Table 13.1   Causes of Hypotension

Rate Problems
   Too slow (Figure 13.5)
      Sinus bradycardia
      Type I and II second-degree heart block
      Third-degree heart block
      Pacemaker failures

   Too fast (Figure 13.6)
      Sinus tachycardia
      Atrial flutter
      Atrial fibrillation
      Paroxysmal supraventricular tachycardia
      Ventricular tachycardia

Pump Problems
   Primary
      Myocardial infarction
      Cardiomyopathies
      Myocarditis
      Ruptured chordae tendineae
      Acute papillary muscle dysfunction
      Acute aortic insufficiency
      Prosthetic valve dysfunction
      Ruptured intraventricular septum

   Secondary
      Drugs that alter function
      Cardiac tamponade
      Pulmonary embolism
      Atrial myxomas
      Superior vena cava syndrome

■ **Table 13.1**   Causes of Hypotension (con't)

Volume Problems
Absolute
Hemorrhage
Gastrointestinal loss
Renal losses
Insensible losses
Adrenal insufficiency (aldosterone)
Relative (vasodilation or redistribution)
Central nervous system injury
Spinal injury
Third-space loss
Tension pneumothorax
Adrenal insufficiency (cortisol)
Sepsis
Drugs that alter vascular tone

Reproduced with permission. CPR Issue, JAMA, October 28, 1992. © American Heart Association.

Rate Problems

1. If a significant rate problem exists and it is unclear whether it is a pump or a volume problem, then treat the heart rate first.
2. Rate problems are not always synonymous with conducting problems. Investigate the underlying etiology.

Volume Problems

1. Volume problems are treated with either fluid (to increase volume) or vasopressors (to increase vascular tone).
2. The first priority is to provide adequate volume.
3. For hypovolemic and hemorrhagic shock, fluid replacement is the treatment of choice. Aim for optimal preload volumes (pulmonary wedge of 12 mm Hg to 15 mm Hg).

Pump Problems

1. It is important to determine the specific cause of the pump failure before instituting treatment.
2. Pump failure may also require treatment for a coexisting rate or volume problem.

Post-Resuscitation Care

Key Points

- Always ensure that appropriate airway control and ventilation continue with required oxygen supplementation during all transfers.
- Rule out any common complications of emergency resuscitation:
  1. Pneumothorax
  2. Pericardial tamponade
  3. Rib fractures
  4. Poorly positioned ET tubes
  5. Bleeding secondary to central line placement attempts
- Check to see that all IV and central line accesses are working properly with the correct fluid/medications (e.g., lidocaine or bretylium) ordered. Replace lines that were inserted without sterile techniques.
- Arrange transfer of resuscitated patients to an appropriate intensive care setting.
- Order all indicated laboratory tests not already drawn, including
  1. Electrolytes
  2. Glucose
  3. CPK-MB (serial measurements will be needed)
  4. Calcium
  5. Magnesium
  6. Arterial blood gases (unless thrombolytic therapy is anticipated)
  7. Blood urea nitrogen
  8. Serum creatinine
- Order a 12-lead ECG if not already done.
- Monitor vital signs on a regular basis and especially during transfer.
- Order a chest x-ray if not done.
- Monitor urine output and record.
- During patient transfers, always have resuscitation equipment accompany the patient with ACLS-trained personnel present.
- Consider thrombolytic therapy for all suspected or confirmed acute MI patients.

Death and Grieving

Dealing with death from unsuccessful resuscitation attempts is difficult for team members and the family. Contact with family members should be done as early as possible with as much information given as known. The inappropriate delivery of information, including the perception by family members that it is being delivered in an uncaring manner, can have long-lasting psychological effects on the survivors.

As most health-care providers do not receive formal training in conveying bad news to others, it is critical that proper time and methods be used in talking with family members.

Key Points

- The person briefing the family should have the most current information and fully understand the events surrounding the emergency as much as possible.
- Always relate to the family the exact circumstances regarding what has transpired in the emergency department setting and be prepared to repeat information as requested.
- Always encourage the family to ask questions and make sure they know how to contact someone later on (even days later) in case questions arise. The personal family attending physician should also be contacted by the emergency department personnel.
- The family should be allowed to see their relative and they should be oriented to what they will be seeing when they enter the room.
- Try to have clergy or social worker present, even if the family has not specifically asked for this.

It can be extremely unsettling for some health-care professionals to convey the news that someone has had an unexpected death. Table 13.2 lists the AHA recommendations for conveying the news of a sudden death to family members.

■ **Table 13.2**   **Conveying News of a Sudden Death to Family Members**

Call the family if they have not been notified. Explain that their loved one has been admitted to the emergency department and that the situation is serious. Survivors should not be told of the death over the telephone.

Obtain as much information as possible about the patient and the circumstances surrounding the death. Carefully go over the events as they happened in the emergency department.

Ask someone to take family members to a private area. Walk in, introduce yourself, and sit down. Address the closest relative.

Briefly describe the circumstances leading to the death. Go over the sequence of events in the emergency department. Avoid euphemisms such as "he's passed on," "she's no longer with us," or "he's left us." Instead, use the words "death," "dying," or "dead."

Allow time for the shock to be absorbed. Make eye contact, touch, and share. Convey your feelings with a phrase such as "You have my (our) sincere sympathy" rather than "I (we) am sorry."

Allow as much time as necessary for questions and discussion. Go over the events several times to make sure everything is understood and to facilitate further questions.

Allow the family the opportunity to see their relative. If equipment is still connected, let the family know.

Know in advance what happens next and who will sign the death certificate. Physicians may impose burdens on staff and family if they fail to understand policies about death certification and disposition of the body. Know the answers to these questions before meeting the family.

Enlist the aid of a social worker or the clergy if not already present.

Offer to contact the patient's attending or family physician and to be available if there are further questions. Arrange for follow-up and continued support during the grieving period.

Critical Incident Debriefing

Team members may have very strong emotional reactions to unsuccessful codes. Interventions to help with these feelings may be very important to prevent personnel from suffering from psychological dysfunction or subsequent burnout. Critical incident debriefings are extremely useful to constructively diffuse or dissipate some of the stress of dealing with emergencies on a regular basis. These debriefings should be held as soon as possible after the event. A separate post-resuscitation *critique* to discuss techniques and other technical matters can be held separately 24 to 72 hours later when any emotional reactions have hopefully been dealt with by team members.

Table 13.3 lists the AHA recommendations for critical incident debriefings.

Table 13.3   **Recommendations for Critical Incident Debriefing**

The debriefing should occur as soon as possible after the event, with all team members present.
Call the group together, preferably in the resuscitation room. State that you want to have a "code debriefing."
Review the events and conduct of the code. Include the contributory pathophysiology leading to the code, the decision tree followed, and any variations.
Analyze the things that were done wrong and especially the things that were done right. Allow free discussion.
Ask for recommendations/suggestions for future resuscitative attempts.
All team members should share their feelings, anxieties, anger, and possible guilt.
Team members unable to attend the debriefing should be informed of the process followed, the discussion generated, and the recommendations made.
The team leader should encourage team members to contact him or her if questions arise later.

Reproduced with permission. CPR Issue. JAMA, October 28, 1992. © American Heart Association.

Notes

14 Case Presentations

Objectives

1. Relate AHA guidelines to specific teaching case scenarios.
2. Identify *key actions* that are required in specific code situations.

The following case scenarios each present a specific situation asking you to describe what key actions you would initiate based on the information presented and your knowledge of ACLS. The suggested responses then follow on the subsequent pages.

Case 1 | Respiratory Arrest

Prehospital

You are called to the fifth-floor walk-up of a building where you find a 38-year-old male in a bathtub of cold water and ice cubes. Bystanders state they tried to bring him "out of it" by giving him large quantities of milk and submerging him in cold water. After removing the person from the tub, you discover that he is apneic.

Emergency Department

A 58-year-old female is transported to the Emergency Department (ED) by taxicab. As she is assisted from a wheelchair to a stretcher you notice that she is not breathing. Her sister, who accompanied her to the ED, states that it has become progressively more difficult for the patient to "catch her breath" over the course of the day. She further states that when her breathing became a problem in the past she would start to take her water pill again.

Hospital

A 55-year old male patient was admitted for respiratory distress secondary to severe chronic obstructive pulmonary disease two days ago. The patient was recently complaining of discomfort and was placed on a non-rebreather at 12 L/min. As you arrive at his bedside to replace his IV, you note the patient is no longer breathing.

What Key Actions Must You Initiate?

_____

_____

_____

_____

_____

_____

_____

_____

_____

_____

_____

Let's See How Well You Have Performed. Did You...

- Ensure use of universal precautions
- Check for responsiveness
- Open airway and assess respirations
- In the absence of respirations, initiate rescue breathing
- Check pulses; if present, continue respiratory support with consideration for identifying problems
- Ensure presence of necessary equipment (airway tray/kit, defibrillator, BVM, oxygen)
- Utilize airway adjuncts (oral airway, ventilate via BVM with supplemental oxygen via reservoir)
- Intubate patient and assess proper placement by listening for bilateral lung sounds and listen for abdominal sounds to ensure that the tube is not in the esophagus with resonant lung sounds (consider use of carbon dioxide sensing cap device)
- Establish IV access
- Evaluate the patient's overall condition
- Arrange for transfer of patient to appropriate intensive care unit and ensure proper ventilatory support and resuscitation equipment during transportation

Don't Let the Following Apply to You!

- Fail to utilize universal precautions
- Perform inadequate/incomplete patient assessment
- Assume and initiate CPR prior to assessing pulses
- Fail to use supplemental oxygen with appropriate device (e.g., oxygen reservoir)
- Fail to check on proper placement of the ET tube or not correct a recognized problem such as a right mainstem intubation
- Use inappropriate intubation technique; fail to hyperventilate prior to intubation or take too much time without stopping to re-ventilate the patient

Summary

It must be recognized that the patient is in respiratory compromise/arrest. Once the patient's respiratory status is appropriately assessed, prompt intervention must occur to correct this condition. The assessment must then continue to pulses and other clinical indicators. As no spontaneous return of respirations occurs, advanced airway support (intubation) is *immediately* initiated and IV access obtained.

| Case 2 | # Ventricular Fibrillation |

Prehospital

You respond to the home of a 52-year-old female. The husband states that while his wife was engaged in strenuous physical activity she developed chest pain with difficulty breathing. He is relieved to see you, as just a moment before you rang the doorbell she stopped answering his questions and closed her eyes.

Emergency Department

A 55-year-old male arrives in the ED by private transport. He states that he developed chest pain and cold sweats while driving his sanitation truck. While undressing, he states he feels nauseous and promptly begins vomiting. After evacuating the contents of his stomach, he collapses back onto the stretcher and loses consciousness.

Hospital

Friends of a 27-year-old male patient who was admitted to the hospital for surgery on a dislocated shoulder frantically request you come to the patient's room. They state they brought the patient a little cocaine to help "cheer him up," but after three or four lines he began to shake and roll his eyes. Upon your arrival, the patient is unconscious.

What Key Actions Must You Initiate?

_____

_____

_____

_____

_____

_____

_____

_____

_____

_____

_____

_____

_____

Let's See How Well You Have Performed. Did You...

- Ensure use of universal precautions
- Check for responsiveness
- Open airway and assess respirations
- In the absence of respirations, support ventilation through rescue breathing
- Check pulses; if absent, begin CPR and call for monitor/defibrillator
- Ensure presence of necessary equipment (airway tray/kit, defibrillator, oxygen)
- Utilize airway adjuncts as indicated/required (oral airway, ventilate via BVM with supplemental oxygen via reservoir) for ventilatory support; intubate as required
- Apply monitor and be able to recognize VF
- Deliver all defibrillatory shocks at proper energy levels

- Use proper safety techniques while delivering defibrillations
- Recognize any changes in rhythm, assess pulses, and, if present, assess other clinical indicators
- Maintain required ventilatory support and airway maintenance during the post-resuscitation period
- Establish IV access and utilize appropriate pharmacology
- Arrange for transfer of patient to appropriate intensive care unit and ensure proper ventilatory support and resuscitation equipment during transportation

Don't Let the Following Apply to You!

- Fail to utilize universal precautions
- Perform inadequate/incomplete patient assessment
- Fail to initiate CPR
- Fail to use supplemental oxygen with appropriate device (e.g., oxygen reservoir)
- Order intubation, IV, or medication administration prior to assessing for the presence of VF and/or prior to attempting defibrillation
- Unable to recognize VF
- Use unsafe technique for delivery of defibrillation (including injury to yourself or other code team members)
- Fail to recognize changes in rhythm and/or lack of pulse assessment
- Fail to maintain ventilatory support and airway maintenance during the post-resuscitation period

Summary

These patients all had witnessed cardiac arrests and, as such, have the greatest opportunity for resuscitation if CPR and prompt defibrillation are performed correctly. Recognition of VF and the primary focus on rapid defibrillation are key to these patients surviving.

| Case 3 | ## Pulseless Electrical Activity |

Prehospital

You are called to the apartment of a 58-year-old male. The room-mate greets you as you enter the elevator to ascend to the 17th floor. The patient's roommate states his friend has been complaining of stomach pain with associated vomiting and frequent bowel move-ments for the past two weeks. Upon arrival at the patient's side, you observe a male lying prone on the living room floor. He is unconscious and lying in a pool of vomitus the consistency of coffee grounds and there is a foul odor in the room.

Emergency Department

A 27-year-old female is transported to the ED by ambulance. She has been in a motor vehicle crash and is fully immobilized on a backboard with high-flow oxygen being delivered via a nonrebreather mask. The EMTs state she has developed increased dyspnea during transportation. The patient is now unconscious.

Hospital

You are called to the room of a 33-year-old female who is com-plaining of chest pain accompanied by dyspnea. She was readmitted early that morning to correct postsurgical complications from a long-bone fracture. Past medical history reveals she smoked cigarettes for the last 10 years but quit six weeks ago. Her only medications are Tylenol #3 (codeine) and birth control pills. As you are obtaining this history, the patient becomes unconscious.

What Key Actions Must You Initiate?

_____

_____

_____

_____

_____

_____

_____

_____

_____

_____

_____

_____

Let's See How Well You Have Performed. Did You...

- Ensure use of universal precautions
- Check for responsiveness
- Open airway and assess respirations
- In the absence of respirations, support ventilation through rescue breathing
- Check pulses; if absent, begin CPR and call for monitor/defibrillator
- Ensure presence of necessary equipment (airway tray/kit, defibrillator, oxygen)
- Utilize airway adjuncts as indicated/required (oral airway, ventilate via BVM with supplemental oxygen via reservoir) for ventilatory support
- Apply monitor and be able to recognize PEA
- Intubate patient and assess proper placement by listening for bilateral lung sounds and listen for abdominal sounds to ensure the

tube is not in the esophagus with resonant lung sounds (consider use of carbon dioxide sensing cap device)

- Establish IV access
- Properly assess the patient and understand the possible underlying causes for PEA, such as hypovolemia, hypoxia, cardiac tamponade, tension pneumothorax, hemothorax (posttraumatic), massive pulmonary embolism, drug overdose (e.g., tricyclics, digoxin, beta blockers, calcium channel blockers), hyperkalemia, pre-existing acidosis, massive anterior wall myocardial infarction, and severe hypothermia
- Recognize any changes in rhythm, assess pulses, and, if present, assess other clinical indicators.

Don't Let the Following Apply to You!

- Fail to utilize universal precautions
- Perform inadequate/incomplete patient assessment (avoid focusing on respiratory problems alone to the exclusion of pulse checks and underlying etiology of respiratory distress)
- Fail to initiate CPR
- Fail to use supplemental oxygen with appropriate device (e.g., oxygen reservoir)
- Unable to recognize PEA
- Fail to order or perform required intubation and/or establish IV access
- Fail to consider the possible causes of PEA
- Fail to consider volume infusions and/or treat only with epinephrine

Summary

The patient is found to be in PEA. This condition may have occurred due to any of the causes previously noted. The patient's presenting condition and available history are critical in determining an appropriate course of action.

Case 4	# Asystole

Prehospital

You are called to the home of a 77-year-old female. Her daughter greets you at the door and states that she returned late last night from a three-day business trip and her mother was sleeping soundly in bed. Upon awakening this morning, she was unable to arouse her mother. In the master bedroom you discover the patient supine on the bed, covered with a large quantity of blankets and quilts. She is unconscious.

Emergency Department

A 23-year-old female was picked up from outside the ED entrance by security. The officer states a car drove into the emergency area, opened the rear door, and ejected the patient. The car promptly sped off. The patient is unconscious and is incontinent of feces and urine. There is evidence of a copious amount of vomitus on her clothing.

Hospital

You are summoned to the room of a 68-year-old male transferred to the floor from intensive care. Upon arrival, you discover the patient in a chair slumped over his food tray. He is having agonal respirations.

What Key Actions Must You Initiate?

_____

_____

_____

_____

_____

_____

_____

_____

Let's See How Well You Have Performed. Did You...

- Ensure use of universal precautions
- Check for responsiveness
- Open airway and assess respirations
- In the absence of respirations, support through rescue breathing
- Check pulses; if absent, begin CPR and call for monitor/defibrillator
- Ensure presence of necessary equipment (airway tray/kit, defibrillator, oxygen)
- Utilize airway adjuncts (oral airway, ventilate via BVM with supplemental oxygen via reservoir) for ventilatory support
- Apply monitor and be able to recognize and confirm asystole in more than one lead
- Intubate patient and assess proper placement by listening for bilateral lung sounds and listen for abdominal sounds to ensure the tube is not in the esophagus with resonant lung sounds (consider use of carbon dioxide sensing cap device)
- Establish IV access
- Recognize the critical role ventilatory support plays in acid-base balance
- Recognize that transcutaneous pacing (TCP) needs to be considered early and concurrent with pharmacology
- Recognize any changes in rhythm, assess pulses, and, if present, assess other clinical indicators

Don't Let the Following Apply to You!

- Fail to utilize universal precautions
- Perform inadequate/incomplete patient assessment
- Fail to initiate CPR
- Fail to use supplemental oxygen with appropriate device (e.g., oxygen reservoir)
- Inability to recognize and confirm asystole in more than one lead
- Fail to order or perform intubation and/or establish IV access
- Fail to consider TCP early or the use of TCP without pharmacologic intervention

Summary

The successful resuscitation of the asystolic patient lies in identifying a treatable cause. Asystole most often represents an indication of death as opposed to a treatable rhythm. Primary considerations for differential diagnosis include adequate ventilatory support to ensure acid-base balance and appropriate and timely use of TCP.

Case 5 — Acute Cardiac Events

Prehospital

You are called to the dining area of a popular dance hall. Upon arrival, you are introduced to a 53-year-old male who is complaining of substernal chest pain that began during a rousing rendition of the hedge hog hop. He notes associated complaints of dyspnea and nausea and says his jaw and left arm also hurt.

Emergency Department

A 66-year-old female is brought to the ED by a friend. The friend states that the patient passed out twice while waiting in line for tickets to a popular Broadway show but refused to go to the hospital until the tickets were acquired. Upon questioning the patient, she feels weak and is ready to vomit. Her skin is cool, pale, and diaphoretic, and she is complaining of an uneasy feeling in her chest.

Hospital

A 43-year-old male who was admitted to the hospital for elective surgery calls you to his room. He states that while watching a hockey game on TV he began to "feel funny." Currently, he is in moderate respiratory distress and complains of severe pain in his chest. He further states he has a family history of "heart problems."

What Key Actions Must You Initiate?

_____

_____

_____

_____

_____

_____

_____

_____

_____

_____

Let's See How Well You Have Performed. Did You...

- Ensure use of universal precautions
- Assess airway, breathing, and circulation (ABCs), and proceed with appropriate action
- Perform a rapid evaluation of the patient inclusive of 12-lead ECG and recognize the ECG criteria for identification of an acute MI
- Initiate oxygen therapy
- Establish IV access
- Perform complete physical exam and obtain history and vital signs
- Know the actions, indications, and contraindications of the pharmacology used in the treatment and care of an acute MI
- Pharmacologic therapy

Don't Let the Following Apply to You!

- Fail to utilize universal precautions
- Fail to thoroughly evaluate the patient's condition inclusive of 12-lead ECG, physical exam, and history
- Fail to initiate appropriate oxygen and pharmacologic therapy
- Administer any medications that are contraindicated for patient condition/status
- Fail to establish IV access

Summary

The patient suffering an acute MI requires prompt assessment, diagnosis, and treatment. Early consideration for use of thrombolytics as well as other pharmacology is essential.

Hypotension/Shock/Pulmonary Edema

Prehospital

You are called to the home of a 54-year-old male. The dispatch information states the caller has some mild difficulty in breathing but seemed anxious. After some difficulty (and delay), you locate the patient's home in a trailer park. Upon entering, you observe the patient sitting in a chair leaning forward breathing noisily. There are open beer cans and empty potato chip bags strewn about the room. The patient is cool, pale, diaphoretic, and anxious.

Emergency Department

A 35-year-old male is transported to the ED by private conveyance. He states that while eating a stuffed sea scroll appetizer in the Sun Cloud Imperial Seafood Emporium he began to feel strange. A friend who drove him to the ED states that his friend passed out for a while. Currently, his skin is red and flushed and he is experiencing mild dyspnea.

Hospital

A 66-year-old male patient is found in his room leaning forward on the side of his bed. He is complaining of weakness and dyspnea. His history is that he was admitted for surgery to correct a gastrointestinal problem. He is lethargic and states he needs to go to the bathroom. As you call for assistance, he begins to slump toward the floor.

What Key Actions Must You Initiate?

_____

_____

_____

_____

_____

_____

_____

_____

_____

_____

_____

_____

Let's See How Well You Have Performed. Did You...

- Ensure use of universal precautions
- Assess ABCs and proceed with appropriate action
- Perform a rapid evaluation of the patient inclusive of 12-lead ECG
- Administer oxygen
- Establish IV access
- Perform complete physical exam, and obtain history and vital signs
- Be observant of all clinical indicators
- Evaluate underlying cause: rate, pump, or volume problem
- Focus therapy on specific system(s) failure as identified
- Be prepared to treat the patient in whom multiple therapeutics will be necessary

Don't Let the Following Apply to You!

- Fail to utilize universal precautions
- Fail to thoroughly evaluate the patient's condition inclusive of 12-lead ECG, physical exam, history, and other clinical indicators

- Fail to initiate appropriate oxygen, IV, and pharmacologic therapies
- Fail to recognize and treat underlying causes or take inappropriate corrective action (e.g., fluid challenge to correct heart rate in strictly rate-related problems)
- Administer morphine sulfate or nitroglycerin to patients in a hypotensive state

Summary

In order to have the best opportunity for survival, these patients require prompt assessment, diagnosis, and treatment. Aggressive airway management, IV therapies, and pharmacology are essential elements of care. Focus on the underlying cause and develop therapeutic strategies based on that problem.

| Case 7 | # Cardiac Arrest Secondary to Drowning |

Prehospital

You are called to a recreational park campsite. Upon arrival, you find a 37-year-old male who was whitewater rafting when he fell from the raft into the water. Witnesses state that he was under a whirlpool for about three minutes. When he surfaced, he was dragged to shore. There is no evidence of gross trauma outwardly visible.

Emergency Department

You are in the nurses' station in the ED when your attention is called to the waiting area where a loud commotion is taking place. Upon investigation, you discover a male carrying a small child dripping wet. As you lead them to a room, the man states that he found the child submerged in his backyard duck pond. It is unknown how long he was under water.

Hospital

A 47-year-old female patient is found submerged in a whirlpool bath. The attendant states that he was away from the area only a short while to go to the bathroom down the hall. The patient was in rehabilitation for a recent sports injury.

What Key Actions Must You Initiate?

_____

_____

_____

_____

_____

_____

_____

_____

_____

_____

_____

_____

_____

_____

Let's See How Well You Have Performed. Did You...

- Ensure use of universal precautions
- Check for responsiveness
- Open airway and assess respirations
- In the absence of respirations, initiate rescue breathing
- Check pulses; if absent, begin CPR and call for monitor/defibrillator

- Ensure presence of necessary equipment (airway tray/kit, defibrillator, oxygen)
- Utilize airway adjuncts (oral airway, ventilate via BVM with supplemental oxygen via reservoir) for ventilatory support
- Apply monitor and be able to recognize the rhythm
- Intubate patient and assess proper placement by listening for bilateral lung sounds and listen for abdominal sounds to ensure the tube is not in the esophagus with resonant lung sounds (consider use of carbon dioxide sensing cap device)
- Establish IV access
- Recognize any changes in rhythm, assess pulses, and, if present, assess other clinical indicators

Don't Let The Following Apply To You!

- Fail to utilize universal precautions
- Perform inadequate/incomplete patient assessment
- Fail to initiate CPR
- Fail to use supplemental oxygen with appropriate device (e.g., oxygen reservoir)
- Unable to recognize ECG rhythm
- Fail to order or perform intubation and/or establish IV access
- Fail to recognize changes in rhythm, assess pulses, and, if present, assess other clinical indicators

Summary

The immediate goal of care with the submersion victim is to evaluate ABCs and provide CPR (with consideration for possible hypothermia). In addition, a major consideration should be spinal immobilization (especially in diving or shallow water incidents). Emphasis is also placed on post-resuscitative care with a focus on the possibility of the patient developing respiratory problems.

Case 8	# Hypothermia

Prehospital

You are called to the bridle path of a local park in the early morning hours of June. You are met by the police who state they have the patient located and are "flushing" him out. They state he is the same fellow they saw last night drinking wine and chased into the woods but could not find. It has rained overnight. As you discuss the case with the police, the patient appears dressed only in underpants and covered with dirt and dried leaves. He is incoherent and his axillae are cold to the touch.

Emergency Department

A police cruiser brings a 32-year-old male into the ED. He was found sleeping on a cardboard box over a defunct heat grid. He is confused and rambling about how hot it is outside and questions why he is being held prisoner. He is immediately recognized by other staff members who state that he has a history of substance abuse and a seizure disorder.

Hospital

A 66-year-old female from the psychiatric ward of the local hospital was found wandering in the snow outside the hospital. The security people stated that she was reportedly missing for about 2 to 3 hours. She appears acutely confused with irregular pulse and skin extremely cold to the touch. She then becomes unconscious with loss of all vital signs.

What Key Actions Must You Initiate?

_____

_____

_____

_____

_____

_____

Let's See How Well You Have Performed. Did You...

- Ensure use of universal precautions
- Assess ABCs and proceed with appropriate action
- Recognize the signs and symptoms of hypothermia
- Give the dead the benefit of the doubt when in deep hypothermia (they may not be dead despite the usual clinical signs of death when hypothermic and must always be assessed for the possibility of rewarming)
- Provide proper temperature monitoring of the patient using low-temperature sensing devices
- ECG Monitor
- Prevent further heat loss: Remove wet garments, cover with blankets, and protect from wind chill
- Administer oxygen (warmed and humidified if possible)
- Gentle handling and transport (horizontally to avoid any orthostatic BP declines)
- Provide gentle airway control; intubate if necessary to secure patient's airway and ventilate with warm, humidified oxygen
- Establish IV (peripherally may not be possible due to vasoconstriction, may need to have central line access when appropriate personnel present) and infuse warm fluids
- Determine medical history of preexisting and associated disease factors (consider presence of drugs, especially alcohol, that the patient may have ingested)
- Avoid external rewarming; it is not done when the patient is in cardiovascular collapse

Don't Let the Following Apply to You!

- Fail to utilize universal precautions
- Allow the hypothermic patient to be declared "cold and dead" without proper assessment for rewarming
- Fail to remove wet garments and protect from wind chill effects
- Fail to deliver warmed, humidified oxygen to the hypothermic patient
- Administer repeated doses of cardiovascular pharmacology to patients in cardiac arrest with a core temperature of <30° C

- Fail to recognize the importance of underlying disease entities, including concurrent drug use
- Fail to practice gentle handling of hypothermic patients in all aspects of care
- Fail to avoid external rewarming (e.g., warming blankets, heating lamps, warm enemas/nasogastric lavage) in patients with cardiac arrest

Summary

The essentials to appropriate patient care center on recognition of hypothermia and patient assessment (responsiveness/level of consciousness). In addition, special consideration must be given to gentle handling during transportation and treatment modalities. The need for appropriate equipment such as electrical/rectal thermometer and probe, needle sensors for ECG as well as devices for active rewarming must also be considered.

Case 9	**Traumatic Cardiac Arrest**

Prehospital

You are called to the scene of a motor vehicle crash. Upon arrival, you find a 57-year-old male lying on the ground next to an auto that has sustained significant front-end and side damage. There is a one-foot intrusion of the left front door into the driver's compartment and the steering wheel has been pushed back toward the seat. A witness states that the driver was sideswiped by a truck and then exited the shoulder of the highway before striking a lamppost. The state police are doing CPR at this time.

Emergency Department

A 28-year-old male is taken to the ED by ambulance. The accompanying police officer states that the patient was earlier forcefully enter-

ing an apartment through a fourth floor window when he lost his grip
and fell three stories (about 30 feet) to the ground. He has been appar-
ently unconscious since the fall, and CPR was initiated when EMS personnel arrived at the scene some four minutes later.

Hospital

A 32-year-old male victim of a gunshot wound is being transported
to the operating room. While on the elevator, he becomes extremely
combative. Shortly thereafter, he lays back on the stretcher exhibiting
agonal respirations.

What Key Actions Must You Initiate?

_____

_____

_____

_____

_____

_____

_____

_____

_____

_____

_____

_____

_____

_____

_____

_____

_____

_____

Let's See How Well You Have Performed. Did You...

- Ensure use of universal precautions
- Check for responsiveness
- Open airway and assess respirations
- In the absence of respirations, initiate rescue breathing
- Check pulses; if absent, begin CPR and call for monitor/defibrillator
- Ensure presence of necessary equipment (airway tray/kit, defibrillator, oxygen)
- Utilize airway adjuncts (oral airway, ventilate via BVM with supplemental oxygen via reservoir) for ventilatory support
- Consider/observe C-spine precautions
- Apply monitor and be able to recognize the rhythm; consider defibrillation for VF as trauma may be secondary to sudden cardiac arrest
- Intubate patient and assess proper placement by listening for bilateral lung sounds and listen for abdominal sounds to ensure the tube is not in the esophagus with resonant lung sounds (consider use of carbon dioxide sensing cap device)
- Establish IV access; utilize appropriate pharmacologic therapy
- Recognize any changes in rhythm, assess pulses, and, if present, assess other clinical indicators
- Consider transport to appropriate trauma care facility

Don't Let the Following Apply to You!

- Fail to utilize universal precautions
- Perform inadequate or incomplete patient assessment
- Fail to initiate CPR
- Fail to use supplemental oxygen with appropriate device (e.g., oxygen reservoir)
- Unable to recognize ECG rhythm or treat VF (recognize its possibility as the precipitating event to trauma)
- Fail to order or perform intubation (with consideration for C-spine precautions) and/or establish IV access
- Fail to recognize changes in rhythm, assess pulses, and, if present, assess other clinical indicators

Summary

Consideration must be given to the fact that the trauma may have occurred secondary to sudden cardiac arrest and, as such, VF should be defibrillated. Information referencing mechanism of injury and patient history may be useful in determining the chronology of precipitating events. Definitive trauma care must not be delayed for extensive ACLS efforts.

Case 10	**Bradycardia**

Prehospital

You are called to a well-known uptown restaurant. Upon arrival, you are escorted to the back offices where you find a 57-year-old female complaining of weakness. As a further history is elicited, you hear that while working in the kitchen the patient began to feel dizzy and suddenly vomited into the soup-of-the-day. The patient states that she has had several similar episodes over the last two weeks of a lesser severity.

Emergency Department

A 66-year-old male is brought to the ED by ambulance. The EMTs state that the patient is complaining of generalized weakness since awakening this morning. The patient further states that whenever he tried to sit up he felt as though he would pass out.

Hospital

A 54-year-old female patient sitting in the admitting office with her husband, who is being admitted, begins to complain of mild chest discomfort and lightheadedness. As she rises to go to the water fountain, she collapses back into her chair. She is pale and diaphoretic.

What Key Actions Must You Initiate?

_____

_____

_____

_____

_____

_____

_____

_____

_____

_____

_____

_____

_____

_____

_____

Let's See How Well You Have Performed. Did You...

- Ensure use of universal precautions
- Assess ABCs and proceed with appropriate action
- Perform a rapid evaluation of the patient inclusive of 12-lead ECG and be able to recognize second- and third-degree blocks
- Perform complete physical exam, obtain history and vital signs, and recognize the signs and symptoms of bradycardia
- Establish IV access and initiate oxygen and pharmacologic therapy in appropriate dosages
- Initiate transcutaneous pacing concurrent with pharmacology
- Recognize the need for transvenous pacing after initial stabilization

Don't Let the Following Apply to You!

- Fail to utilize universal precautions
- Fail to thoroughly evaluate the patient's condition inclusive of 12-lead ECG, history, and physical exam
- Fail to recognize the signs and symptoms of bradycardia
- Fail to initiate appropriate oxygen and pharmacologic therapy
- Fail to initiate transcutaneous pacing concurrent with pharmacologic intervention
- Inappropriately administer lidocaine to suppress life-saving escape rhythms
- Inappropriately treat an asymptomatic bradycardic patient
- Fail to recognize the need for transvenous pacing after initial stabilization

Summary

Appropriate management of the patient found to be bradycardic may prevent primary arrest or recurring arrest post-resuscitation. Recognition of the signs and symptoms of bradycardia as well as primary use of pharmacologic treatment and transcutaneous pacing are essential aspects of appropriate care for these patients. Diagnosis of the level and degree of block is important in making the final decision on the need for permanent pacing.

Case 11   Unstable Tachycardia/Electrical Conversion

Prehospital

You are dispatched to the holding cell of the local Transit Authority police station. Upon arrival, you are led to a 52-year-old male complaining of palpitations and who states "I can't catch my wind." He is cool, pale, and diaphoretic, and he states that he is unable to ambulate.

Emergency Department

A 66-year-old female arrives in the ED complaining of a "weird" feeling in her chest accompanied by weakness. She is nauseous and states that if she does not sit down soon she will fall. She is anxious and is constantly patting herself on the sternum.

Hospital

A 67-year-old male, who is visiting a friend who recently had a gall bladder operation, summons you to the patient's room. The man then proceeds to tell you that the patient is OK, but *he* is experiencing severe chest pain with shortness of breath. He states that he was on his way to get his friend a drink of water when he felt as though he would pass out.

What Key Actions Must You Initiate?

_____

_____

_____

_____

_____

_____

_____

_____

_____

_____

_____

_____

_____

_____

Let's See How Well You Have Performed. Did You...

- Ensure use of universal precautions
- Assess ABCs and proceed with appropriate action
- Perform a rapid evaluation of the patient inclusive of 12-lead ECG and be able to recognize VT
- Perform complete physical exam, obtain history and vital signs, and recognize the signs and symptoms of cardiovascular instability
- Deliver synchronized cardioversion in a safe and appropriate manner at the proper energy levels
- Recognize any changes in rhythm and monitor all clinical indicators
- Establish IV access; initiate oxygen and pharmacologic therapy in appropriate dosages
- Recognize the need to progress from synchronized cardioversion for VT to unsynchronized defibrillation anytime VF is identified

Don't Let the Following Apply to You!

- Fail to utilize universal precautions
- Perform inadequate or incomplete patient assessment, physical exam, and identification of underlying etiology
- Fail to use supplemental oxygen with appropriate device (e.g., oxygen reservoir)
- Unable to recognize VT
- Fail to recognize changes in rhythm, apply oxygen, establish IV, and treat with appropriate pharmacology
- Fail to recognize the need to go from synchronized cardioversion to unsynchronized defibrillation should VF develop

Summary

The ventricular tachycardic patient with an unstable cardiovascular system may require synchronized cardioversion. It is important to recognize both the ECG rhythm and the signs and symptoms of instability. In addition, the need for supplemental oxygen and recognition of deterioration to VF must be recognized.

| Case 12 | **Stable Ventricular Tachycardia** |

Prehospital

You are called to the home of a 66-year-old female who collapsed after swimming four laps in her Olympic-size swimming pool. The patient is complaining of chest palpitations.

Emergency Department

A 22-year-old male arrives in the ED complaining of a funny feeling in his chest. He is anxious and complains vehemently about the lack of proper care as he has not yet been examined. He becomes verbally abusive while denying use of any "recreational" drugs, although no one has asked. Blood pressure and pulse are within normal limits.

Hospital

A 70-year-old male, post-appendectomy patient is preparing for discharge. He has been complaining on and off to his wife of a "queasy" feeling in his epigastric region and chest but has found relief by taking a chewable antacid pill. You are summoned to the room by his wife who requests that he be given a "once over" before he leaves. Upon entering the room, you discover the patient standing near the window with his suitcase in hand ready to go home. He does not look well.

What Key Actions Must You Initiate?

_____

_____

_____

_____

_____

_____

_____

_____

Let's See How Well You Have Performed. Did You...

- Ensure use of universal precautions
- Assess ABCs and proceed with appropriate action
- Perform a rapid evaluation of the patient inclusive of 12-lead ECG and be able to recognize VT
- Perform complete physical exam, obtain history and vital signs, and recognize the signs of cardiovascular instability
- Establish IV access; initiate oxygen and pharmacologic therapy in appropriate dosages
- Recognize any changes in rhythm and monitor all clinical indicators
- Be prepared to utilize synchronized cardioversion should physical and pharmacologic interventions be unsuccessful

Don't Let the Following Apply to You!

- Fail to utilize universal precautions
- Perform inadequate or incomplete patient assessment, physical exam, and identification of underlying etiology
- Fail to use supplemental oxygen with appropriate device (e.g., oxygen reservoir)
- Unable to recognize VT
- Utilize unsafe technique for delivery of cardioversion (e.g., shocking yourself, fellow clinicians, or innocent bystanders)
- Fail to recognize changes in rhythm, apply oxygen, establish IV, and/or treat with appropriate pharmacologic intervention
- Fail to recognize the need to go to synchronized cardioversion should other measures fail

Summary

Initial assessment should be achieved quickly to determine the stability or instability of the patient's cardiovascular system. The patient with a relatively stable cardiovascular system may effectively be treated with just pharmacologic intervention. If those measures are unsuccessful, synchronized cardioversion may be required. It is important to recognize both the ECG rhythm and the signs and symptoms of instability. In addition, the need for supplemental oxygen and monitoring of clinical indicators must occur.

ACLS Practice ECG Test

ACLS ECG Practice Test Answer Sheet

Directions: Enter the letter preceding the ECG strips on the following pages in the blank corresponding to the correct rhythm description. One answer for each and no answer is ever repeated.

_____ Course VF

_____ Sinus tachycardia

_____ Atrial flutter with 4:1 block

_____ Unifocal PVCs with couplets

_____ Second-degree AV block (Mobitz I)

_____ Atrial fibrillation

_____ Sinus bradycardia with premature atrial contractions

_____ Ventricular tachycardia

_____ Third-degree AV block (complete heart block)

_____ 60-Hz artifact

_____ Unifocal PVCs

_____ Sinus rhythm into a PSVT

_____ Second-degree AV block (Mobitz II)

_____ Ventricular paced rhythm

_____   Agonal rhythm (dying heart)

_____   Sinus rhythm

_____   Junctional rhythm

_____   Multifocal PVCs

_____   First-degree AV block

_____   Asystole

A.

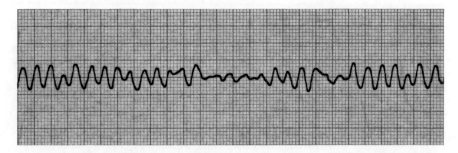

B.

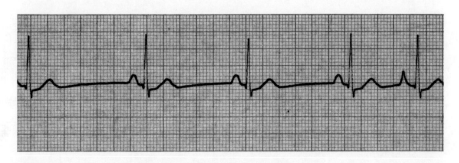

C.

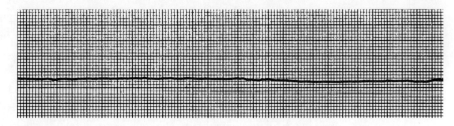

D.

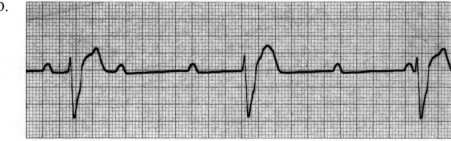

E.

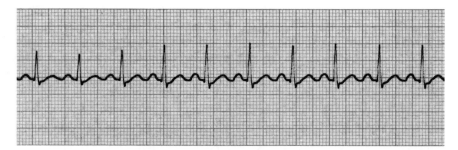

F.

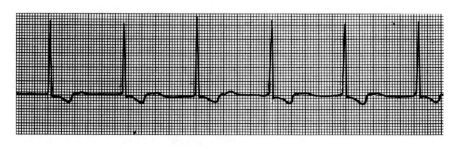

G.

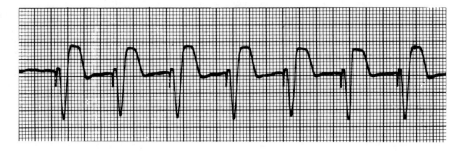

H.

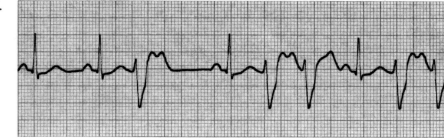

I.

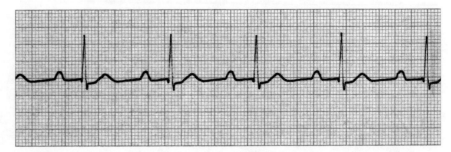

J.

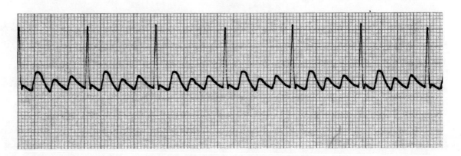

K.

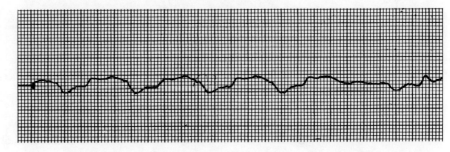

L.

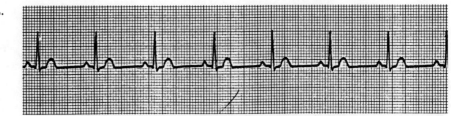

M.

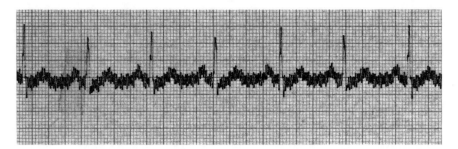

N.

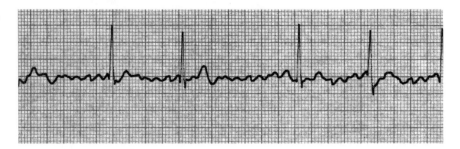

O.

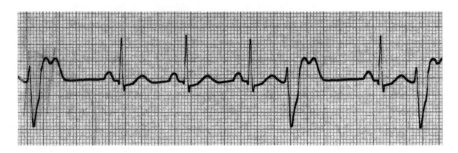

P.

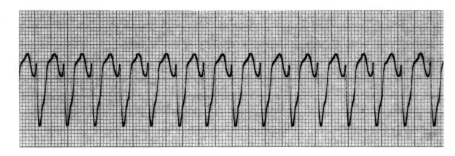

Q.

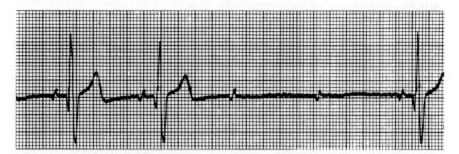

R.

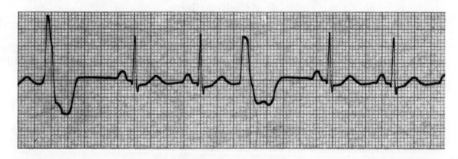

S.

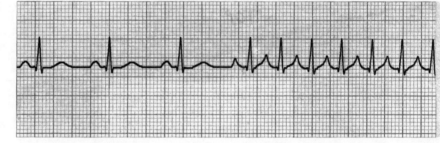

T.

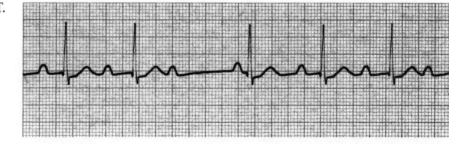

Answer Key:
ACLS ECG Practice Test Answer Sheet

A   Coarse VF
E   Sinus tachycardia
J   Atrial flutter with 4:1 block
H   Unifocal PVCs with couplets
T   Second-degree AV block (Mobitz I)
N   Atrial fibrillation
B   Sinus bradycardia with premature atrial contractions
P   Ventricular tachycardia
D   Third-degree AV block (complete heart block)
M   60-Hz artifact
O   Unifocal PVCs
S   Sinus rhythm into a PSVT
Q   Second-degree AV block (Mobitz II)
G   Ventricular paced rhythm
K   Agonal rhythm (dying heart)
L   Sinus rhythm
F   Junctional rhythm
R   Multifocal PVCs
I   First-degree AV block
C   Asystole

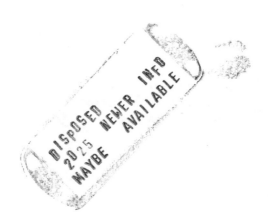

ACLS Practice Exam Questions

Directions: Pick the one best answer and place this answer on the answer sheet found on p 212.

1. Which drug should *not* be used for a patient in cardiogenic pulmonary edema whose vital signs are P=124, BP 108 systolic, and an ECG that indicates a sinus tachycardia?

   a. Furosemide
   b. Atropine
   c. Oxygen
   d. Morphine

2. In a patient who has suffered an MI, the ECG will always be abnormal.

   a. True
   b. False

3. Automated external defibrillator pads (electrodes) should be placed over the apex of the heart (left midaxillary line) and the upper chest just right of the sternum.

   a. True
   b. False

4. Successful completion of an ACLS provider course implies that the individual is "licensed" by the AHA to perform ACLS.

   a. True
   b. False

5. A 72-year-old female patient is delivered to the hospital ED by a basic life support ambulance. Upon admission to the ED, her vital signs are recorded and indicate the following: P=50, BP=60/40. The ECG indicates a first-degree heart block with ventricular ectopy. Which is the first-line drug of choice?

   a. Isoproterenol
   b. Lidocaine
   c. Verapamil
   d. Atropine

6. The most common initial misplacement of the ET tube, resulting in minimal breath sounds and poor blood gases, is generally caused by the ET tube being inserted into the

   a. Left mainstem bronchus
   b. Trachea
   c. Right mainstem bronchus
   d. Esophagus

7. Once the determination has been made that an unwitnessed cardiac arrest patient is in VF, the next immediate course of action is to

   a. Perform an ET intubation
   b. Administer epinephrine IV or via the ET tube
   c. Defibrillate at 200 J
   d. Perform a precordial thump

8. The most accessible vein to cannulate initially while performing CPR on a patient is

   a. Antecubital
   b. Saphenous
   c. Internal jugular
   d. Femoral

9. While treating a patient in the ED or ambulance who you suspect has suffered an MI, you begin to witness what you interpret as numerous multiform ventricular ectopic beats. Within the next minute, the patient becomes unconscious and pulseless, and the monitor shows VF. Your next immediate course of action is to

   a. Perform CPR
   b. Perform an ET intubation
   c. Perform a precordial thump
   d. Administer lidocaine

10. A 44-year-old male patient arrives in the employee health unit complaining of jaw pain and a dull pressure in his left arm. At this time, the patient is conscious and alert but experiencing some dif-

ficulty breathing. After placing the patient on a monitor, you notice that the rhythm indicates what looks like a narrow-complex tachycardia with a rate of approximately 160 and a BP of 100/68. Your next course of action is to

   a. Administer verapamil at a dose of 20 mg IV push
   b. Perform carotid sinus massage to see effect on rate
   c. Administer lidocaine immediately
   d. Perform synchronized cardioversion after sedation

11. All automated external defibrillators can perform simultaneous ECG interpretation while CPR is being performed on the patient.

   a. True
   b. False

12. Ventricular fibrillation is the most common rhythm seen in the first minute following a cardiac arrest.

   a. True
   b. False

13. The diagnosis of acute MI is based primarily on the ECG.

   a. True
   b. False

14. The most important treatment for correcting acidosis during a cardiac arrest is to

   a. Administer sodium bicarbonate
   b. Perform CPR
   c. Ventilate with 100% oxygen
   d. Administer calcium chloride

15. Suctioning the patient requires that this procedure be performed while the suction catheter is being withdrawn from the oropharynx.

   a. True
   b. False

16. A 77-year-old female patient has just been admitted to the cardiac care unit (CCU) as a rule-out MI. The patient states that she has been experiencing severe chest discomfort that is crushing in nature. Prior to arriving at the ED, she had taken four nitroglycerin tablets with no relief. Her past medical history indicates that she has angina and hypertension for which she is being treated by her family physician. Her vital signs are as follows: P=98, BP=104/72, and her ECG reveals a normal sinus rhythm. What is the best initial course of treatment?

a. Atropine
b. Morphine
c. Lasix
d. Lidocaine

17. The acidosis that usually occurs during cardiac arrest is treated by proper ventilation of the victim.

a. True
b. False

18. Synchronized cardioversion is the initial treatment of choice for

a. Ventricular fibrillation
b. Asystole
c. Unstable ventricular tachycardia
d. Sinus tachycardia

19. Which drug cannot be administered via the transtracheal route?

a. Lidocaine
b. Epinephrine
c. Morphine
d. Narcan

20. Atropine 1.0 mg

a. May not be administered via the transtracheal route
b. Is the recommended initial dose for asystole
c. May cause transient tachycardia if administered slowly
d. Can be repeated no more than three times

21. For which of the following patients would ET intubation be the preferred method of airway management?

    a.   Conscious patient with a suspected third-degree AV block
    b.   Unconscious patient with an intact airway
    c.   Stable patient with ventricular ectopy
    d.   Unconscious patient with an unstable airway

22. You are presented with an 80-kg male patient who has suffered a cardiac arrest. The ECG reveals that the patient is in VF. Your initial defibrillation attempt was unsuccessful at 200 J. What would the next energy setting be for defibrillation?

    a.   50 to 80 J
    b.   80 to 100 J
    c.   200 to 300 J
    d.   360 to 400 J

23. Endotracheal intubation should be performed ideally in less than 30 seconds.

    a.   True
    b.   False

24. Nitroglycerin

    a.   Should be administered via the transtracheal route
    b.   Should be limited to two doses sublingually
    c.   May produce hypertension
    d.   May be helpful in relieving pain from an MI

25. The dosage for transtracheal drug administration is usually

    a.   The same as the IV dose
    b.   One to one and one-half times the IV dose
    c.   Two to two and one-half times the IV dose
    d.   Three times the IV dose

26. Which of the following is expected to *not* assist in decreasing transthoracic resistance during defibrillation?

    a. Multiple countershocks
    b. Use of conductive gel
    c. Minimal paddle pressure
    d. Proper placement of the paddles

27. Dopamine administered in low doses of 2 to 5 μg/kg/min will result in renal vasodilatation.

    a. True
    b. False

28. Identify the following dysrhythmia:

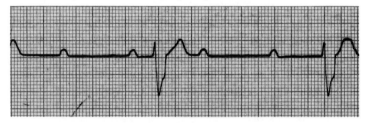

    a. Sinus bradycardia
    b. Second-degree type I AV block
    c. Third-degree AV block
    d. Second-degree type II AV block

29. Identify the following dysrhythmia:

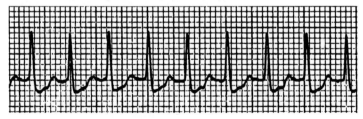

    a. Sinus tachycardia
    b. Ventricular tachycardia
    c. Atrial fibrillation
    d. Supraventricular tachycardia

30. Identify the following dysrhythmia:

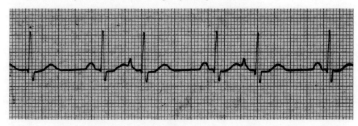

   a. Third-degree AV block
   b. Sinus rhythm with premature atrial contractions
   c. Second-degree type I AV block
   d. Second-degree type II AV block

31. Which of the following is *not* an indication for stopping the administration of procainamide?

   a. Hypotension develops
   b. The QRS complex widens by 50% or more
   c. Hypertension develops
   d. One to two grams total have been administered

32. Which ECG rhythm is most likely to be seen in patients who have suffered a significant electrical shock?

   a. Ventricular tachycardia
   b. Sinus rhythm with ectopy
   c. Ventricular asystole
   d. Ventricular fibrillation

33. For trauma patients who are presenting with PEA, which of the following conditions will most likely *not* be a contributing factor?

   a. Hypotension
   b. Tension pneumothorax
   c. Alkalosis
   d. Hypovolemia

34. Verapamil facilitates successful electrical conversion from VF to a viable rhythm.

    a.   True
    b.   False

35. Which drug administered in correct doses will increase myocardial contractility?

    a.   Lidocaine
    b.   Epinephrine
    c.   Propranolol
    d.   Verapamil

36. A 62-year-old woman has been picked up by the mobile intensive care unit with the primary chief complaint being "a syncopal episode." Upon examination, the paramedic notices that the patient has an irregular pulse, and the ECG reveals sinus rhythm with multiformed ventricular beats occurring and a short run of VT. What is the most likely initial course of treatment that will be approved by the physician medical command?

    a.   Lidocaine infusion
    b.   Atropine
    c.   Propranolol
    d.   Lidocaine bolus

37. Ventricular fibrillation can be mimicked by artifact on the ECG monitor.

    a.   True
    b.   False

38. Cardiopulmonary resuscitation has been initiated on a patient in asystole. The first drug of choice would be

    a.   Sodium bicarbonate
    b.   Epinephrine
    c.   Calcium chloride
    d.   Verapamil

39. Verapamil would be the first drug of choice for a pulseless patient whose ECG reveals narrow-complex tachycardia with P waves preceding each QRS complex. The rate is approximately 120.

 a. True
 b. False

40. The drug of choice for terminating PSVT is

 a. Adenosine
 b. Lidocaine
 c. Bretyllium
 d. Verapamil

41. The paramedic unit arrives in the ED with a 32-year-old male who has fallen 40 feet from a scaffold. The patient's vital signs are P=134, BP=60/40, R=36. The patient's skin color is ashen and pulses are absent in the periphery. The treatment of choice is

 a. Fluid replacement
 b. Vasopressors
 c. Vasodilators
 d. External pacing

42. A 35-year-old woman who is seven months pregnant has suffered a cardiac arrest. The patient's ECG reveals VF. Which one of the following treatments should be accomplished?

 a. Avoid all medication use
 b. Do not shift the uterus off of the vena cava during CPR
 c. Never allow a cesarean section
 d. Treat according to the VF algorithm

43. A 66-year-old male has been admitted to the CCU with a rule-out MI. The patient is now presenting as somewhat lethargic with pallor. In addition, the patient is diaphoretic and has a pulse of 200. When you auscultate the BP, the readings indicate 70/50. The ECG reveals a supraventricular tachycardia. The first intervention should be

a. Propranolol
b. Procainamide
c. Verapamil
d. Synchronized cardioversion

44. During the course of treating a patient with synchronized cardioversion, the patient develops pulseless VF. The next step is to increase the J level and deliver another synchronized cardioversion shock.

a. True
b. False

45. Bag-valve-mask airway management devices should only be used by individuals trained in their use.

a. True
b. False

46. Endotracheal suctioning should be limited to

a. Five seconds
b. Ten seconds
c. Fifteen seconds
d. There is no limit

47. Sodium bicarbonate therapy

a. May be administered at anytime during the code situation
b. Does not require constant blood gas analysis for use
c. May cause metabolic alkalosis
d. Should be added to IV solutions containing catecholamines

48. Electrical defibrillation is the preferred initial method of treatment for patients who have suffered a cardiac arrest.

    a. True
    b. False

49. Isoproterenol has all of the following actions except

    a. Increased force of contraction
    b. Increased heart rate
    c. Alpha-adrenergic stimulation
    d. Increased myocardial irritability

50. If you had a choice of any of the following, which would you choose?

    a. Take an ACLS course
    b. Go on a vacation
    c. Read another textbook

Practice Exam Questions Answer Sheet

Place the correct answer in the space provided.

1. _____	21. _____	41. _____
2. _____	22. _____	42. _____
3. _____	23. _____	43. _____
4. _____	24. _____	44. _____
5. _____	25. _____	45. _____
6. _____	26. _____	46. _____
7. _____	27. _____	47. _____
8. _____	28. _____	48. _____
9. _____	29. _____	49. _____
10. _____	30. _____	50. _____
11. _____	31. _____	
12. _____	32. _____	
13. _____	33. _____	
14. _____	34. _____	
15. _____	35. _____	
16. _____	36. _____	
17. _____	37. _____	
18. _____	38. _____	
19. _____	39. _____	
20. _____	40. _____	

Practice Exam Questions Answer Key

1. B	21. D	41. A
2. B	22. C	42. D
3. A	23. A	43. D
4. B	24. D	44. B
5. D	25. C	45. A
6. C	26. C	46. C
7. C	27. A	47. C
8. A	28. C	48. B
9. C	29. D	49. C
10. B	30. B	50. B
11. B	31. C	
12. A	32. D	
13. B	33. C	
14. C	34. B	
15. A	35. B	
16. B	36. D	
17. A	37. A	
18. C	38. B	
19. C	39. B	
20. B	40. A	

Rationale For Answers

1. **B** Atropine will increase the heart rate, which could further lower the systolic pressure. The increased heart rate is an attempt by the body to increase pressure by increasing the rate. Affecting the rate in this clinical situation would have serious consequences. All the other medications are appropriate.

2. **B** The ECG may be entirely normal in a patient having an MI.

3. **A** Automated external defibrillator electrodes are placed in the same position as are the defibrillator paddles:
   a. Right midclavicular line just below clavicle
   b. Left midaxillary line at about the 6th rib level

4. **B**   Passing ACLS means that the individual on a given day passed the minimal material required for its standards. It is not a "certification" or a "license," implying that the individual will always be performing ACLS correctly in the future.

5. **D**   The heart rate is slow with a subsequent decrease in BP and the ventricular ectopy being an escape rhythm. If the rate is increased through the use of atropine, it should help resolve at least the hypotension.

6. **C**   Intubation of the right mainstem bronchus often occurs due to the anatomical positioning of the opening of the right mainstem bronchus before the left mainstem bronchus.

7. **C**   Defibrillation is the only definitive treatment for VF and the sooner it is performed the greater is the chance of converting it to a more normal, life-sustaining rhythm.

8. **A**   The antecubital vein is the most accessible and safest to cannulate during CPR.

9. **C**   A precordial thump is performed only in a witnessed, monitored situation for VF or unstable VT. If unsuccessful, proceed immediately to electrical therapy, if a defibrillator is available, or start CPR.

10. **B**   The only correct answer with the choices given is to perform carotid sinus massage and assess the effect on the rate. All of the other choices are inappropriate in this clinical setting.

11. **B**   Cardiopulmonary resuscitation must be stopped while the AEDs are performing ECG interpretation and/or defibrillating, as the CPR may cause interference.

12. **A**   Upwards of 80% to 90% of cardiac arrest victims are found to be in VF.

13. **B**   The diagnosis of an MI is also made taking into consideration the patient's clinical presentation and history.

14. **C**   The easiest and safest way to prevent or correct acidosis is with adequate and proper oxygenation. If sodium bicarbonate is administered indiscriminately the patient may become alkalotic, which presents another problem.

15. **A**   Suctioning is performed only while the catheter is being withdrawn so as not to deprive the patient any further of necessary oxygen.

16. **B** The use of morphine will treat not only the pain and reduce anxiety but also provide an increase in venous capacitance, thus decreasing venous return. This will be useful in the treatment of pulmonary edema. It can also cause a mild arterial vasodilation.

17. **A** Respiratory acidosis is the primary cause of the acidosis seen during cardiac arrest. Ventilation or hyperventilation is the primary modality of treatment.

18. **C** If the patient is unstable (e.g., hypotensive, angina, pulmonary edema) he or she is in need of more definitive treatment than medication, and synchronized cardioversion is the treatment choice for VT with a pulse.

19. **C** All the drugs listed can be given via the transtracheal route except morphine.

20. **B** Atropine in a dose of 1.0 mg is the initial recommended dose for asystole.

21. **D** If the patient is showing severe signs of decompensation (such as being unconscious and with respiratory difficulty), he or she will most likely require continued airway support. The airway can be better maintained and with improved oxygenation for the patient once intubation is performed.

22. **C** There are two schools of thought concerning this issue. Some believe the transthoracic resistance decreases with subsequent electrical shocks and would recommend the use of 200 J for the second shock. Others think the transthoracic resistance is decreased so minimally with subsequent shocks that it is best to increase the J level to 300 for the second time. The best answer of those given is 200 to 300 J for the second shock.

23. **A** Ventilation should not be interrupted for more than 30 seconds at a time, including during intubation attempts.

24. **D** Nitroglycerin relaxes vascular smooth muscle resulting in dilation of both venous and arterial blood vessels. Left ventricular preload and afterload are reduced and myocardial oxygen consumption or demand is decreased. Collateral circulation in MI patients is improved and blood flow to ischemic areas is increased. Answer D is the only correct answer.

25. **C** In general, drugs administered via the transtracheal route should be given at two to two and one-half the usual IV dose.

26. **C** Good, firm paddle pressure (approximately 25 lbs) will decrease the transthoracic resistance.

27. **A** Dopamine in a dose of 2 to 5 μg/kg/min will result in mainly renal vasodilation. At a range of 2 to 10 μg/kg/min this will also cause an increased cardiac output.

28. **C** The rhythm is third-degree block since there is no relationship between the P waves and the QRS complexes.

29. **D** The rhythm shown is a supraventricular tachycardia.

30. **B** All the beats look the same (sinus in nature), but some are premature. The best answer is a sinus rhythm with premature atrial contractions.

31. **C** Procainamide has the potential to cause hypotension, *not* hypertension.

32. **D** Ventricular fibrillation is the most common dysrhythmia seen in patients who have undergone a significant electrical shock.

33. **C** Alkalosis is not a major cause of PEA.

34. **B** Verapamil may facilitate a decrease in heart rate by inhibiting calcium ion influx into the cells of the myocardial muscle. As a result, intracellular calcium remains at subthreshold levels insufficient to stimulate cell excitation and contraction. It also decreases and slows SA and AV node conduction. But it has no capabilities of actually converting VF to normal sinus rhythm.

35. **B** Epinephrine, when ordered correctly, will increase myocardial contractility.

36. **D** Given the clinical situation presented, a bolus of lidocaine would be the most likely initial order.

37. **A** Ventricular fibrillation can be mimicked by artifact or even a disconnected lead and, therefore, clinical assessment is required for all patients thought to be in VF.

38. **B** Epinephrine is beneficial for the reason that it increases coronary blood flow and automaticity, thereby, helping to restore a cardiac rhythm with subsequent increases in BP, heart rate, and myocardial contractility. This is the correct initial drug of choice in asystole.

39. **B** Given this clinical scenario, being that the patient is *pulseless*, the initial management is not to give verapamil. The diagnosis is probably PEA.

40. **A** Adenosine is now the drug of choice for terminating PSVT.

41. **A** Given the history of a fall with hypotension, a secondary tachycardia, and no obvious signs of external blood or fluid loss, there must be internal bleeding. First, stabilize the patient with fluid replacement and then look for the source of the blood loss.

42. **D** The only correct choice is treatment according to the VF algorithm. All the other choices listed are incorrect.

43. **D** The patient is clearly unstable (with signs of lethargy, increased heart rate, decreased blood pressure) but with an organized rhythm (with QRS complexes), so proceed with the most definitive treatment, which is *synchronized cardioversion*.

44. **B** Once the patient has developed VF, you can no longer use synchronized cardioversion because there is no R wave for the defibrillator to sense. The correct answer would be to *defibrillate* the patient with 200 J.

45. **A** Only trained individuals would have the ability to effectively oxygenate during a BVM system.

46. **C** The 15-second limit is used so as not to deprive the patient of needed oxygen any longer than is absolutely necessary.

47. **C** A metabolic alkalosis may develop if it is given indiscriminately without the benefit of blood gas analysis. All of the other answers are incorrect.

48. **B** You first need to know what rhythm the patient's heart is in before determining your choice of therapy. Not all cardiac arrest patients are in VF.

49. **C** Isoproterenol is a pure beta-adrenergic agonist. All of the other answers are correct.

50. **B** Don't be a fool—relax, enjoy yourself, and go on vacation!!!!! (You've earned it, haven't you!!!)

Notes

Index

Notes

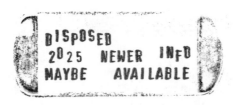

Easy ACLS Quick Reference Chart 1

BCLS Performance Guidelines

	Infant (≤ 1 Year)	Child (1 to 8 Years)	Adult
Airway	Head tilt/chin lift (If trauma suspected, jaw thrust)	Same	Same
Breathing	2 breaths at 1 to 1½ sec/breath	Same	2 breaths at 1½ to 2 sec/breath
Compress with	2 fingers	Heel of 1 hand	2 hands (heel) stacked
Position	1 finger's width below intermammary line	Locate end of sternum with middle finger, index finger next to it, heel of hand beside it	Same (except heel of other hand beside it and stack hands)
Depth of compression	½ to 1 inch	1 to 1½ inches	1½ to 2 inches
Pulse check	Brachial	Carotid	Carotid
Rate of compression	At least 100/min	100/min	80 to 100/min
Ratio of compressions to ventilations	5:1	5:1	15:2 (1-person CPR) 5:1 (2-person CPR)
Rescue breathing	1 breath every 3 sec (20 per min)	Same	1 breath every 5 to 6 sec (10 to 12 per min)
Foreign-body airway obstruction	Back blows and chest thrusts	Abdominal thrusts	Same

From *Easy ACLS: Advanced Cardiac Life Support Preparatory Manual* by Andrew D. Weinberg and James L. Paturas. Copyright © 1995 by Jones and Bartlett Publishers, Inc.

Easy ACLS Quick Reference Chart 2

ACLS Algorithms

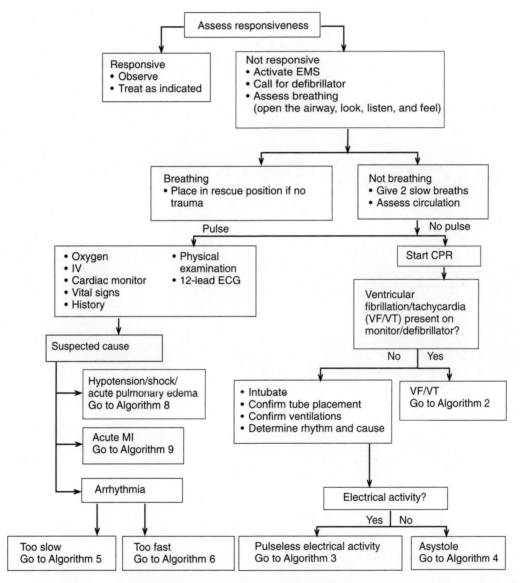

Algorithm 1   Universal algorithm for adult emergency cardiac care (ECC). Reproduced with permission. CPR Issue, JAMA, October 28, 1992. © American Heart Association.

From *Easy ACLS: Advanced Cardiac Life Support Preparatory Manual* by Andrew D. Weinberg and James L. Paturas. Copyright © 1995 by Jones and Bartlett Publishers, Inc.

ACLS Algorithms

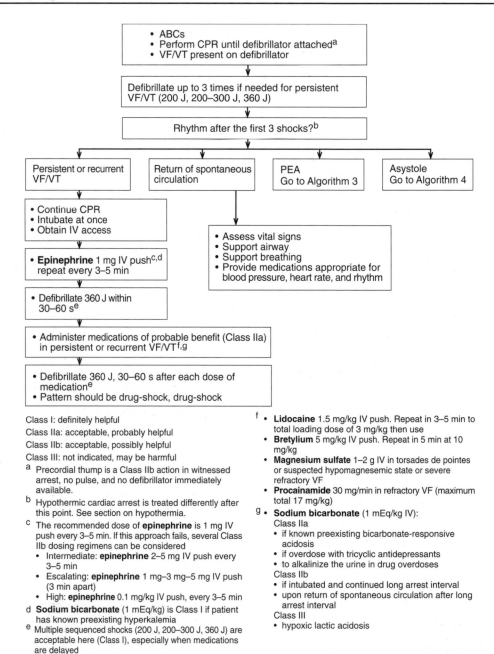

- ABCs
- Perform CPR until defibrillator attached[a]
- VF/VT present on defibrillator

↓

Defibrillate up to 3 times if needed for persistent VF/VT (200 J, 200–300 J, 360 J)

↓

Rhythm after the first 3 shocks?[b]

| Persistent or recurrent VF/VT | Return of spontaneous circulation | PEA Go to Algorithm 3 | Asystole Go to Algorithm 4 |

Persistent or recurrent VF/VT

- Continue CPR
- Intubate at once
- Obtain IV access

↓

- **Epinephrine** 1 mg IV push[c,d] repeat every 3–5 min

↓

- Defibrillate 360 J within 30–60 s[e]

↓

- Administer medications of probable benefit (Class IIa) in persistent or recurrent VF/VT[f,g]

↓

- Defibrillate 360 J, 30–60 s after each dose of medication[e]
- Pattern should be drug-shock, drug-shock

Return of spontaneous circulation

- Assess vital signs
- Support airway
- Support breathing
- Provide medications appropriate for blood pressure, heart rate, and rhythm

---

Class I: definitely helpful
Class IIa: acceptable, probably helpful
Class IIb: acceptable, possibly helpful
Class III: not indicated, may be harmful

a Precordial thump is a Class IIb action in witnessed arrest, no pulse, and no defibrillator immediately available.

b Hypothermic cardiac arrest is treated differently after this point. See section on hypothermia.

c The recommended dose of **epinephrine** is 1 mg IV push every 3–5 min. If this approach fails, several Class IIb dosing regimens can be considered
  - Intermediate: **epinephrine** 2–5 mg IV push every 3–5 min
  - Escalating: **epinephrine** 1 mg–3 mg–5 mg IV push (3 min apart)
  - High: **epinephrine** 0.1 mg/kg IV push, every 3–5 min

d **Sodium bicarbonate** (1 mEq/kg) is Class I if patient has known preexisting hyperkalemia

e Multiple sequenced shocks (200 J, 200–300 J, 360 J) are acceptable here (Class I), especially when medications are delayed

f
- **Lidocaine** 1.5 mg/kg IV push. Repeat in 3–5 min to total loading dose of 3 mg/kg then use
- **Bretylium** 5 mg/kg IV push. Repeat in 5 min at 10 mg/kg
- **Magnesium sulfate** 1–2 g IV in torsades de pointes or suspected hypomagnesemic state or severe refractory VF
- **Procainamide** 30 mg/min in refractory VF (maximum total 17 mg/kg)

g
- **Sodium bicarbonate** (1 mEq/kg IV):
  Class IIa
  - if known preexisting bicarbonate-responsive acidosis
  - if overdose with tricyclic antidepressants
  - to alkalinize the urine in drug overdoses
  Class IIb
  - if intubated and continued long arrest interval
  - upon return of spontaneous circulation after long arrest interval
  Class III
  - hypoxic lactic acidosis

Algorithm 2 Algorithm for ventricular fibrillation and pulseless ventricular tachycardia (VF/VT). Reproduced with permission. CPR Issue, JAMA, October 28, 1992. © American Heart Association.

PEA includes
- Electromechanical dissociation (EMD)
- Pseudo-EMD
- Idioventricular rhythms
- Ventricular escape rhythms
- Bradyasystolic rhythms
- Postdefibrillation idioventricular rhythms

- Continue CPR
- Intubate at once
- Obtain IV access
- Assess blood flow using Doppler ultrasound

↓

Consider possible causes (Parentheses = possible therapies and treatments)
- Hypovolemia (volume infusion)
- Hypoxia (ventilation)
- Cardiac tamponade (pericardiocentesis)
- Tension pneumothorax (needle decompression)
- Hypothermia (see Algorithm 11)
- Massive pulmonary embolism (surgery, **thrombolytics**)
- Drug overdoses such as tricyclics, digitalis, ß-blockers, calcium channel blockers
- Hyperkalemia [a]
- Acidosis [b]
- Massive acute myocardial infarction (go to Algorithm 9)

↓

- **Epinephrine** 1 mg IV push,[a,c] repeat every 3–5 min

↓

- If absolute bradycardia (<60 beats/min) or relative bradycardia, give **atropine** 1 mg IV
- Repeat every 3–5 min up to a total of 0.04 mg/kg[d]

Class I: definitely helpful
Class IIa: acceptable, probably helpful
Class IIb: acceptable, possibly helpful
Class III: not indicated, may be harmful

[a] **Sodium bicarbonate** 1 mEq/kg is Class I if patient has known preexisting hyperkalemia.

[b] **Sodium bicarbonate** 1 mEq/kg:
Class IIa
- if known preexisting bicarbonate-responsive acidosis
- if overdose with tricyclic antidepressants
- to alkalinize the urine in drug overdoses
Class IIb
- if intubated and long arrest interval
- upon return of spontaneous circulation after long arrest interval

Class III
- hypoxic lactic acidosis

[c] The recommended dose of **epinephrine** is 1 mg IV push every 3–5 min. If this approach fails, several Class IIb dosing regimens can be considered.
- Intermediate: **epinephrine** 2–5 mg IV push every 3–5 min
- Escalating: **epinephrine** 1 mg-3 mg-5 mg IV push (3 min apart)
- High: **epinephrine** 0.1 mg/kg IV push every 3–5 min

[d] Shorter **atropine** dosing intervals are possibly helpful in cardiac arrest (Class IIb)

Algorithm 3 Algorithm for pulseless electrical activity (PEA) (electromechanical dissociation [EMD]). Reproduced with permission. CPR Issue, JAMA, October 28, 1992. © American Heart Association.

From *Easy ACLS: Advanced Cardiac Life Support Preparatory Manual* by Andrew D. Weinberg and James L. Paturas. Copyright © 1995 by Jones and Bartlett Publishers, Inc.

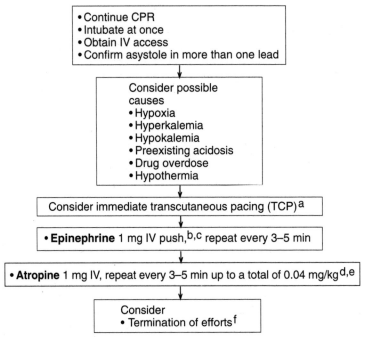

- Continue CPR
- Intubate at once
- Obtain IV access
- Confirm asystole in more than one lead

Consider possible causes
- Hypoxia
- Hyperkalemia
- Hypokalemia
- Preexisting acidosis
- Drug overdose
- Hypothermia

Consider immediate transcutaneous pacing (TCP) [a]

- **Epinephrine** 1 mg IV push,[b,c] repeat every 3–5 min

- **Atropine** 1 mg IV, repeat every 3–5 min up to a total of 0.04 mg/kg [d,e]

Consider
- Termination of efforts [f]

Class I: definitely helpful

Class IIa: acceptable, probably helpful

Class IIb: acceptable, possibly helpful

Class III: not indicated, may be harmful

[a] TCP is a Class IIb intervention. Lack of success may be due to delays in pacing. To be effective TCP must be performed early, simultaneously with drugs. Evidence does not support routine use of TCP for asystole.

[b] The recommended dose of **epinephrine** is 1 mg IV push every 3–5 min. If this approach fails, several Class IIb dosing regimens can be considered:
- Intermediate: **epinephrine** 2–5 mg IV push every 3–5 min
- Escalating: **epinephrine** 1 mg-3 mg-5 mg IV push (3 min apart)
- High: **epinephrine** 0.1 mg/kg IV push every 3–5 min

[c] **Sodium bicarbonate** 1 mEq/kg is Class I if patient has known preexisting hyperkalemia.

[d] Shorter **atropine** dosing intervals are Class IIb in asystolic arrest.

[e] **Sodium bicarbonate** 1 mEq/kg
Class IIa
- if known preexisting bicarbonate-responsive acidosis
- if overdose with tricyclic antidepressants
- to alkalinize the urine in drug overdoses
Class IIb
- if intubated and continued long arrest interval
- upon return of spontaneous circulation after long arrest interval
Class III
- hypoxic lactic acidosis

[f] If patient remains in asystole or other agonal rhythms after successful intubation and initial medications and no reversible causes are identified, consider termination of resuscitative efforts by a physician. Consider interval since arrest.

Algorithm 4   Asystole treatment algorithm. Reproduced with permission. CPR Issue, JAMA, October 28, 1992. © American Heart Association.

ACLS Algorithms

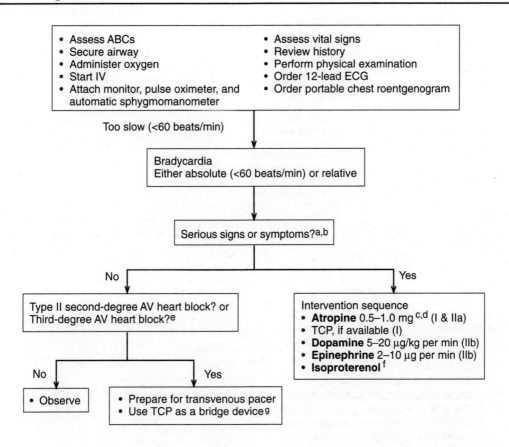

- Assess ABCs
- Secure airway
- Administer oxygen
- Start IV
- Attach monitor, pulse oximeter, and automatic sphygmomanometer

- Assess vital signs
- Review history
- Perform physical examination
- Order 12-lead ECG
- Order portable chest roentgenogram

Too slow (<60 beats/min)

Bradycardia
Either absolute (<60 beats/min) or relative

Serious signs or symptoms?[a,b]

No

Type II second-degree AV heart block? or Third-degree AV heart block?[e]

No — • Observe

Yes — • Prepare for transvenous pacer
• Use TCP as a bridge device[g]

Yes

Intervention sequence
- **Atropine** 0.5–1.0 mg [c,d] (I & IIa)
- TCP, if available (I)
- **Dopamine** 5–20 µg/kg per min (IIb)
- **Epinephrine** 2–10 µg per min (IIb)
- **Isoproterenol** [f]

a Serious signs or symptoms must be related to the slow rate. Clinical manifestations include: *symptoms* (chest pain, shortness of breath, decreased level of consciousness) and *signs* (low BP, shock, pulmonary congestion, CHF, acute MI).

b Do not delay TCP while awaiting IV access or for **atropine** to take effect if patient is symptomatic.

c Denervated transplanted hearts will not respond to **atropine**. Go at once to pacing, **catecholamine** infusion, or both.

d **Atropine** should be given in repeat doses in 3–5 min up to total of 0.04 mg/kg. Consider shorter dosing intervals in severe clinical conditions. It

has been suggested that atropine should be used with caution in atrioventricular (AV) block at the His-Purkinje level (type II AV block and new third-degree block with wide QRS complexes) (Class IIb).

e Never treat third-degree heart block plus ventricular escape beats with **lidocaine**.

f **Isoproterenol** should be used, if at all, with extreme caution. At low doses it is Class IIb (possibly helpful); at higher doses it is Class III (harmful).

g Verify patient tolerance and mechanical capture. Use analgesia and sedation as needed.

Algorithm 5   Bradycardia algorithm (with the patient not in cardiac arrest). Reproduced with permission. CPR Issue, JAMA, October 28, 1992. © American Heart Association.

From *Easy ACLS: Advanced Cardiac Life Support Preparatory Manual* by Andrew D. Weinberg and James L. Paturas. Copyright © 1995 by Jones and Bartlett Publishers, Inc.

ACLS Algorithms

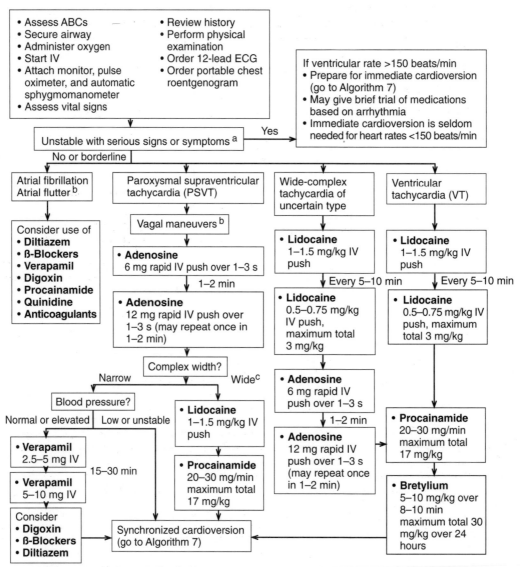

- Assess ABCs
- Secure airway
- Administer oxygen
- Start IV
- Attach monitor, pulse oximeter, and automatic sphygmomanometer
- Assess vital signs

- Review history
- Perform physical examination
- Order 12-lead ECG
- Order portable chest roentgenogram

If ventricular rate >150 beats/min
- Prepare for immediate cardioversion (go to Algorithm 7)
- May give brief trial of medications based on arrhythmia
- Immediate cardioversion is seldom needed for heart rates <150 beats/min

Unstable with serious signs or symptoms [a] — **Yes** →

No or borderline

Atrial fibrillation Atrial flutter [b]

Consider use of
- **Diltiazem**
- **ß-Blockers**
- **Verapamil**
- **Digoxin**
- **Procainamide**
- **Quinidine**
- **Anticoagulants**

Paroxysmal supraventricular tachycardia (PSVT)

Vagal maneuvers [b]

- **Adenosine** 6 mg rapid IV push over 1–3 s

1–2 min

- **Adenosine** 12 mg rapid IV push over 1–3 s (may repeat once in 1–2 min)

Complex width?

Narrow / **Wide [c]**

Blood pressure?

Normal or elevated | **Low or unstable**

- **Verapamil** 2.5–5 mg IV

15–30 min

- **Verapamil** 5–10 mg IV

Consider
- **Digoxin**
- **ß-Blockers**
- **Diltiazem**

Wide-complex tachycardia of uncertain type

- **Lidocaine** 1–1.5 mg/kg IV push

Every 5–10 min

- **Lidocaine** 0.5–0.75 mg/kg IV push, maximum total 3 mg/kg

- **Adenosine** 6 mg rapid IV push over 1–3 s

1–2 min

- **Adenosine** 12 mg rapid IV push over 1–3 s (may repeat once in 1–2 min)

Ventricular tachycardia (VT)

- **Lidocaine** 1–1.5 mg/kg IV push

Every 5–10 min

- **Lidocaine** 0.5–0.75 mg/kg IV push, maximum total 3 mg/kg

- **Procainamide** 20–30 mg/min maximum total 17 mg/kg

- **Bretylium** 5–10 mg/kg over 8–10 min maximum total 30 mg/kg over 24 hours

Wide [c]

- **Lidocaine** 1–1.5 mg/kg IV push

- **Procainamide** 20–30 mg/min maximum total 17 mg/kg

Synchronized cardioversion (go to Algorithm 7)

[a] Unstable condition must be related to the tachycardia. Signs and symptoms may include chest pain, shortness of breath, decreased level of consciousness, low blood pressure (BP), shock, pulmonary congestion, congestive heart failure, acute myocardial infarction.

[b] Carotid sinus pressure is contraindicated in patients with carotid bruits, avoid ice-water immersion in patients with ischemic heart disease.

[c] If the wide-complex tachycardia is known with certainty to be PSVT and BP is normal/elevated, sequence can include **verapamil**.

Algorithm 6   Tachycardia algorithm. Reproduced with permission. CPR Issue, JAMA, October 28, 1992. © American Heart Association.

From *Easy ACLS: Advanced Cardiac Life Support Preparatory Manual* by Andrew D. Weinberg and James L. Paturas. Copyright © 1995 by Jones and Bartlett Publishers, Inc.

ACLS Algorithms

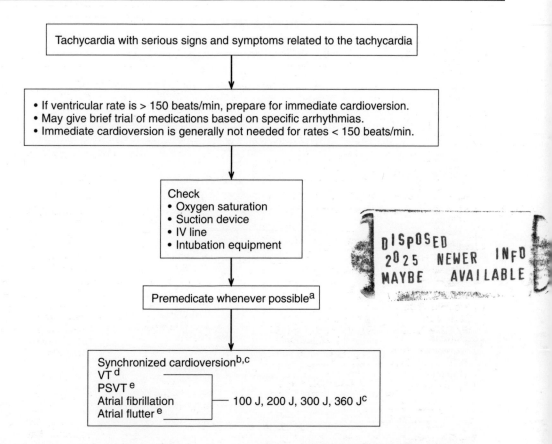

Tachycardia with serious signs and symptoms related to the tachycardia

- If ventricular rate is > 150 beats/min, prepare for immediate cardioversion.
- May give brief trial of medications based on specific arrhythmias.
- Immediate cardioversion is generally not needed for rates < 150 beats/min.

Check
- Oxygen saturation
- Suction device
- IV line
- Intubation equipment

Premedicate whenever possible[a]

Synchronized cardioversion[b,c]
VT [d]
PSVT [e]
Atrial fibrillation ———— 100 J, 200 J, 300 J, 360 J[c]
Atrial flutter [e]

[a] Effective regimens have included a sedative (e.g., **diazepam, midazolam, barbiturates, etomidate, ketamine, methohexital**) with or without an analgesic agent (e.g., **fentanyl, morphine, meperidine**). Many experts recommend anesthesia if service is readily available.
[b] Note possible need to resynchronize after each cardioversion.
[c] If delays in synchronization occur and clinical conditions are critical, go to immediate unsynchronized shocks.
[d] Treat polymorphic VT (irregular form and rate) like VF: 200 J, 200–300 J, 360 J.
[e] PSVT and atrial flutter often respond to lower energy levels (start with 50 J).

Algorithm 7   **Electrical cardioversion algorithm (with the patient not in cardiac arrest). Reproduced with permission. CPR Issue, JAMA, October 28, 1992. © American Heart Association.**

From *Easy ACLS: Advanced Cardiac Life Support Preparatory Manual* by Andrew D. Weinberg and James L. Paturas. Copyright © 1995 by Jones and Bartlett Publishers, Inc.

ACLS Algorithms

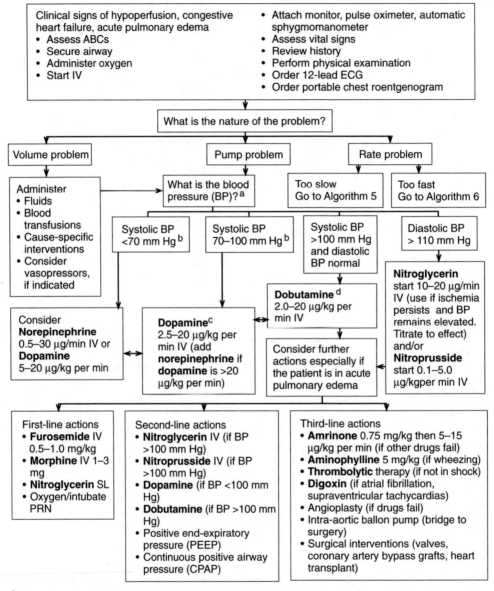

Clinical signs of hypoperfusion, congestive heart failure, acute pulmonary edema
- Assess ABCs
- Secure airway
- Administer oxygen
- Start IV

- Attach monitor, pulse oximeter, automatic sphygmomanometer
- Assess vital signs
- Review history
- Perform physical examination
- Order 12-lead ECG
- Order portable chest roentgenogram

What is the nature of the problem?

Volume problem | **Pump problem** | **Rate problem**

Administer
- Fluids
- Blood transfusions
- Cause-specific interventions
- Consider vasopressors, if indicated

What is the blood pressure (BP)?[a]

Too slow
Go to Algorithm 5

Too fast
Go to Algorithm 6

Systolic BP <70 mm Hg[b]

Systolic BP 70–100 mm Hg[b]

Systolic BP >100 mm Hg and diastolic BP normal

Diastolic BP > 110 mm Hg

Nitroglycerin start 10–20 µg/min IV (use if ischemia persists and BP remains elevated. Titrate to effect) and/or **Nitroprusside** start 0.1–5.0 µg/kg per min IV

Dobutamine[d] 2.0–20 µg/kg per min IV

Consider **Norepinephrine** 0.5–30 µg/min IV or **Dopamine** 5–20 µg/kg per min

Dopamine[c] 2.5–20 µg/kg per min IV (add **norepinephrine** if **dopamine** is >20 µg/kg per min)

Consider further actions especially if the patient is in acute pulmonary edema

First-line actions
- **Furosemide** IV 0.5–1.0 mg/kg
- **Morphine** IV 1–3 mg
- **Nitroglycerin** SL
- Oxygen/intubate PRN

Second-line actions
- **Nitroglycerin** IV (if BP >100 mm Hg)
- **Nitroprusside** IV (if BP >100 mm Hg)
- **Dopamine** (if BP <100 mm Hg)
- **Dobutamine** (if BP >100 mm Hg)
- Positive end-expiratory pressure (PEEP)
- Continuous positive airway pressure (CPAP)

Third-line actions
- **Amrinone** 0.75 mg/kg then 5–15 µg/kg per min (if other drugs fail)
- **Aminophylline** 5 mg/kg (if wheezing)
- **Thrombolytic** therapy (if not in shock)
- **Digoxin** (if atrial fibrillation, supraventricular tachycardias)
- Angioplasty (if drugs fail)
- Intra-aortic balloon pump (bridge to surgery)
- Surgical interventions (valves, coronary artery bypass grafts, heart transplant)

[a] Base management after this point on invasive hemodynamic monitoring if possible.
[b] Fluid bolus of 250–500 mL normal saline should be tried. If no response, consider sympathomimetics.
[c] Move to **dopamine** and stop **norepinephrine** when BP improves.
[d] Add **dopamine** when BP improves. Avoid **dobutamine** when systolic BP <100 mm Hg.

Algorithm 8   Algorithm for hypotension, shock, and acute pulmonary edema. Reproduced with permission. CPR Issue, JAMA, October 28, 1992. © American Heart Association.

From *Easy ACLS: Advanced Cardiac Life Support Preparatory Manual* by Andrew D. Weinberg and James L. Pa.uras. Copyright © 1995 by Jones and Bartlett Publishers, Inc.

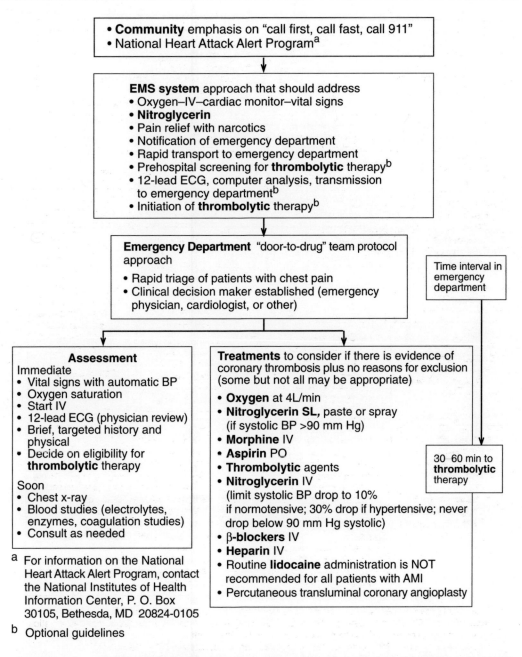

- **Community** emphasis on "call first, call fast, call 911"
- National Heart Attack Alert Program[a]

EMS system approach that should address
- Oxygen–IV–cardiac monitor–vital signs
- **Nitroglycerin**
- Pain relief with narcotics
- Notification of emergency department
- Rapid transport to emergency department
- Prehospital screening for **thrombolytic** therapy[b]
- 12-lead ECG, computer analysis, transmission to emergency department[b]
- Initiation of **thrombolytic** therapy[b]

Emergency Department "door-to-drug" team protocol approach
- Rapid triage of patients with chest pain
- Clinical decision maker established (emergency physician, cardiologist, or other)

Time interval in emergency department

Assessment

Immediate
- Vital signs with automatic BP
- Oxygen saturation
- Start IV
- 12-lead ECG (physician review)
- Brief, targeted history and physical
- Decide on eligibility for **thrombolytic** therapy

Soon
- Chest x-ray
- Blood studies (electrolytes, enzymes, coagulation studies)
- Consult as needed

Treatments to consider if there is evidence of coronary thrombosis plus no reasons for exclusion (some but not all may be appropriate)

- **Oxygen** at 4L/min
- **Nitroglycerin SL,** paste or spray (if systolic BP >90 mm Hg)
- **Morphine** IV
- **Aspirin** PO
- **Thrombolytic** agents
- **Nitroglycerin** IV (limit systolic BP drop to 10% if normotensive; 30% drop if hypertensive; never drop below 90 mm Hg systolic)
- **β-blockers** IV
- **Heparin** IV
- Routine **lidocaine** administration is NOT recommended for all patients with AMI
- Percutaneous transluminal coronary angioplasty

30–60 min to **thrombolytic** therapy

a For information on the National Heart Attack Alert Program, contact the National Institutes of Health Information Center, P. O. Box 30105, Bethesda, MD 20824-0105

b Optional guidelines

Algorithm 9 Acute myocardial infarction (MI) algorithm. Recommendations for early management of patients with chest pain and possible acute MI. Reproduced with permission. CPR issue, JAMA, October 28, 1992. © American Heart Association.

ACLS Algorithms

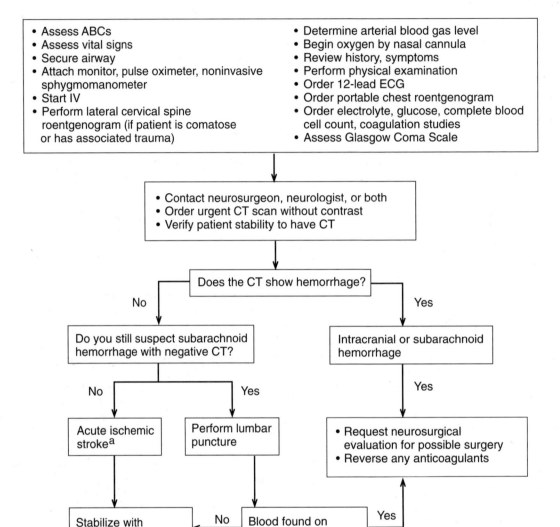

- Assess ABCs
- Assess vital signs
- Secure airway
- Attach monitor, pulse oximeter, noninvasive sphygmomanometer
- Start IV
- Perform lateral cervical spine roentgenogram (if patient is comatose or has associated trauma)

- Determine arterial blood gas level
- Begin oxygen by nasal cannula
- Review history, symptoms
- Perform physical examination
- Order 12-lead ECG
- Order portable chest roentgenogram
- Order electrolyte, glucose, complete blood cell count, coagulation studies
- Assess Glasgow Coma Scale

- Contact neurosurgeon, neurologist, or both
- Order urgent CT scan without contrast
- Verify patient stability to have CT

Does the CT show hemorrhage?

No → Do you still suspect subarachnoid hemorrhage with negative CT?

Yes → Intracranial or subarachnoid hemorrhage

No → Acute ischemic stroke[a]

Yes → Perform lumbar puncture

Yes →
- Request neurosurgical evaluation for possible surgery
- Reverse any anticoagulants

Stabilize with appropriate therapies ← No — Blood found on lumbar puncture? — Yes →

[a] The detailed management of acute stroke is beyond the scope of the ACLS program. Management of cardiovascular emergencies in stroke victims is similar to the management in other patients. Never forget, however, that acute stroke can coexist with acute cardiovascular problems.

Algorithm 10   Algorithm for initial evaluation of suspected stroke. Reproduced with permission. CPR issue, JAMA, October 28, 1992. © American Heart Association.

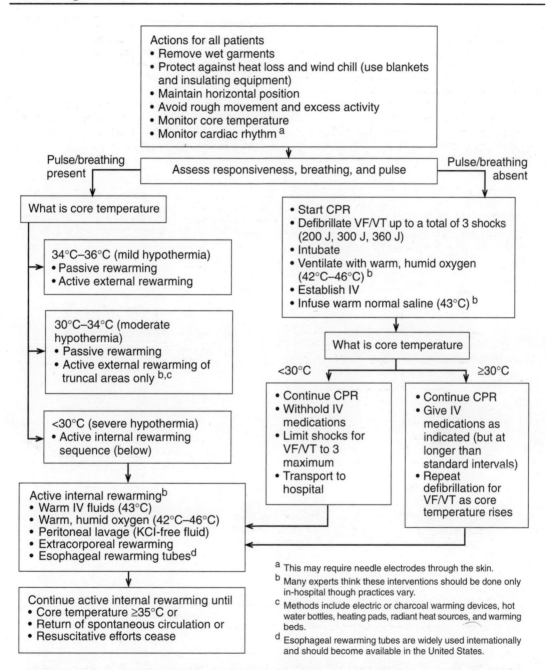

Actions for all patients
- Remove wet garments
- Protect against heat loss and wind chill (use blankets and insulating equipment)
- Maintain horizontal position
- Avoid rough movement and excess activity
- Monitor core temperature
- Monitor cardiac rhythm [a]

Pulse/breathing present

Assess responsiveness, breathing, and pulse

Pulse/breathing absent

What is core temperature

34°C–36°C (mild hypothermia)
- Passive rewarming
- Active external rewarming

30°C–34°C (moderate hypothermia)
- Passive rewarming
- Active external rewarming of truncal areas only [b,c]

<30°C (severe hypothermia)
- Active internal rewarming sequence (below)

- Start CPR
- Defibrillate VF/VT up to a total of 3 shocks (200 J, 300 J, 360 J)
- Intubate
- Ventilate with warm, humid oxygen (42°C–46°C) [b]
- Establish IV
- Infuse warm normal saline (43°C) [b]

What is core temperature

<30°C

- Continue CPR
- Withhold IV medications
- Limit shocks for VF/VT to 3 maximum
- Transport to hospital

≥30°C

- Continue CPR
- Give IV medications as indicated (but at longer than standard intervals)
- Repeat defibrillation for VF/VT as core temperature rises

Active internal rewarming [b]
- Warm IV fluids (43°C)
- Warm, humid oxygen (42°C–46°C)
- Peritoneal lavage (KCl-free fluid)
- Extracorporeal rewarming
- Esophageal rewarming tubes [d]

Continue active internal rewarming until
- Core temperature ≥35°C or
- Return of spontaneous circulation or
- Resuscitative efforts cease

[a] This may require needle electrodes through the skin.

[b] Many experts think these interventions should be done only in-hospital though practices vary.

[c] Methods include electric or charcoal warming devices, hot water bottles, heating pads, radiant heat sources, and warming beds.

[d] Esophageal rewarming tubes are widely used internationally and should become available in the United States.

Algorithm 11   Algorithm for treatment of hypothermia. Reproduced with permission. CPR issue, JAMA, October 28, 1992. © American Heart Association.

From *Easy ACLS: Advanced Cardiac Life Support Preparatory Manual* by Andrew D. Weinberg and James L. Paturas. Copyright © 1995 by Jones and Bartlett Publishers, Inc.

Easy ACLS Quick Reference Chart 3

ACLS Adult Drug Chart

Drug	Use	Dosage	Complications
Adenosine Supplied: 3 mg/mL in 2-mL vials (total = 6 mg)	PSVTs (involving re-entry pathway including AV node)	6 mg rapid IV bolus over 1 s to 3 s. Follow with 20 mL saline flush Repeat with 12-mg rapid IV push if no response within 1 to 2 min	Avoid in second- or third-degree heart block and sick sinus syndrome Dyspnea, flushing, chest pain (all side effects usually resolve within 1 to 2 min) Transient sinus bradycardia or ventricular ectopy may occur after terminating SVT Dipyridamole potentiates its effects Theophylline decreases effects
Amrinone Supplied: 5 mg/mL in 20-mL vials (total =100 mg). Mix in 0.45% normal saline to maximum of 3 mg/mL (750mg/250 mL.)	1. Low cardiac output 2. Refractory CHF	Loading dose: 0.75 mg/kg over 2 to 3 min, followed by infusion of 5 to 15 µg/kg/min	Worsen ventricular ectopy Exacerbate myocardial ischemia
Atropine Supplied: 0.1 mg/mL in 10-mL preloaded syringes (total =1 mg) Can be given via ET tube	1. Sinus bradycardia 2. Asystole 3. AV block at nodal level	Asystole and slow PEA: 1 mg IV and repeat in 3 to 5 min Bradycardia: 0.5 mg to 1.0 mg IV every 3 to 5 min to a total dose of 0.04 mg/kg (= 3 mg*)	Increases myocardial oxygen demands Can increase ischemia or infarction (secondary to excessive increase in rate) Avoid in glaucoma Rare VF/VT with IV use Can trigger tachyarrhythmias and angina *Reserve total vagolytic dose of 3 mg for asystolic arrest

ACLS Adult Drug Chart (continued)

Drug	Use	Dosage	Complications
β-adrenergic blockers Supplied: *Metoprolol:* 1 mg/mL in 5 = mL vials (total = 5 mg). *Atenolol:* 0.5 mg/mL in 10-mL ampules (total = 5 mg) *Propranolol:* 4 mg/mL in 5-mL vials (total = 20 mg)	1. Thrombolytic treated patients (may reduce reinfarction rate and ischemia) 2. Prevent VF in post-MI patients 3. Stable angina	*Atenolol:* 5 mg to 10 mg IV over 5 min *Metoprolol:* 5 mg to 10 mg slow IV push at 5-min intervals until total of 15 mg. *Oral:* 50 mg BID to 100 mg BID after 24 hrs *Propranolol:* total dose of 0.1mg/kg by slow IV push in 3 equal doses at 2 to 3-min intervals (do not exceed rate of 1 mg/min). *Oral:* 180 mg/day to 320 mg/day in divided doses	Hypotension AV conduction delays Bradycardias Decreased myocardial contraction Avoid in patients with asthma/COPD, diabetes, PVD
Bretylium Supplied: 50 mg/mL in 10-mL prefilled syringes (total = 500 mg); 50 mg/mL in 10 = mL vials (total = 500 mg	1. VF and VT after defibrillation, epinephrine, and lidocaine have failed 2. Wide-complex tachycardias unresponsive to lidocaine and adenosine	VF: 5 mg/kg IV bolus. If VF persists, increase to 10 mg/kg and repeat every 5 min up to maximum of 30 mg/kg to 35 mg/kg Recurrent VT: 5 mg/kg to 10 mg/kg diluted in 50 mL D5W IV over 8 to 10 min Infusion: 1 mg/min to 2 mg/min (mix 500 mg in 250 mL of D5W)	Hypotension Bradycardia Nausea and vomiting with rapid IV administration Dizziness/syncope Do not use in known aortic stenosis Use with extreme caution in arrhythmias due to digitalis toxicity
Calcium Supplied: 100 mg/mL in 10 = mL vials (total = 1gm; a 10% solution)	1. Hypocalcemia 2. Calcium channel blocker toxicity 3. Hyperkalemia	10% solution of CaCl in a dose of 2 mg/kg to 4 mg/kg and repeated as necessary at 10-min intervals Ca gluconate in a dose of 5 mL to 8 mL	Hypercalcemia Arrhythmias (e.g., bradycardia, asystole, VF) Extravasation may cause tissue necrosis
Digitalis Supplied: 0.5 mg/2 mL 0.1 mg/1 mL	1. Atrial arrhythmias 2. CHF	Loading dose: 0.5 mg IV or po, followed by 0.25 mg IV/po Q 6H (total dose = 1 mg)	AV block Bradycardia Arrhythmias

From *Easy ACLS: Advanced Cardiac Life Support Preparatory Manual* by Andrew D. Weinberg and James L. Paturas. Copyright © 1995 by Jones and Bartlett Publishers, Inc.

ACLS Adult Drug Chart (continued)

Drug	Use	Dosage	Complications
Digitalis (con't)		For acute suppression of atrial arrhythmias, drug can be given 0.25 mg IV Q 30 to 45 min	Monitor blood levels Avoid hypokalemia
Dobutamine Supplied: 12.5 mg/mL in 20-mL vials (total = 250 mg)	1. Low cardiac output 2. Treatment of heart failure 3. Increase myocardial contractility	Infusion: 2 to 20 µg/kg/min Infusion: Dilute 500 mg to 1,000 mg (40 mL to 80 mL) in 250 mL NS or D5W	Increased heart rate, which may exacerbate ischemia and can cause angina and increased BP PVCs Reflex peripheral vasodilation with secondary hypotension
Dopamine Supplied: 40 mg/mL in 5-mL ampules (total = 200 mg) or 160 mg/mL (total = 800 mg) IV infusion: mix 400 mg to 800 mg in 250 mL NS, LR, or D5W	1. Decreased urine output 2. Low cardiac output 3. Hypotension	Renal dose: 1 to 2 µg/kg/min Increased cardiac output: 2 to 10 µg/kg/min Hypotension: >10 µg/kg/min Infusion: 2.5 to 5 µg/kg/min and titrate to effect	Increased HR Arrhythmias Undesirable degree of vasoconstriction **Do not** use with bicarbonate in same IV line *or* in patients with hypotention secondary to hypovolemia MAO inhibitors potentiate effects of dopamine
Epinephrine Supplied: Preloaded 10-mL syringe: 1 mg/10 mL Glass 1-mL ampule: 1mg/mL Multidose 30-mL vials: 1 mg/mL Can be given via ET tube	1. VF 2. Asystole 3. Symptomatic bradycardia (though not first-line agent)	1.0 mg (10 mL of 1:10,000 solution) IV every 3 to 5 min. Follow with 20 mL flush of IV fluid If this dose fails, 5 mg or 0.1 mg/kg (acceptable, but neither recommended nor discouraged) Infusion: 1 mg (1 mL of 1:1,000 solution) added to 500 mL NS/D5W and given 2 to 10 µg/min Endotracheal: 2 mg to 2.5 mg diluted in 10 mL NS	Increased HR Arrhythmias Ischemia Do not administer in same line as alkaline solutions Peripheral injections should be followed by 20-mL flush of IV fluid to assist with effective distribution of drug Administration for continuous infusions should be through central access to reduce extravasation

From *Easy ACLS: Advanced Cardiac Life Support Preparatory Manual* by Andrew D. Weinberg and James L. Paturas. Copyright © 1995 by Jones and Bartlett Publishers, Inc.

Drug	Use	Dosage	Complications
Furosemide Supplied: 10 mg/mL in ampules Syringes of 2 mL, 4 mL, 10 mL		0.5 mg/kg to 1.0 mg/kg IV slowly *Oral:* 20 mg to 40 mg po initially, increase dose as clinically indicated	Hypotension Hyponatremia Dehydration Hypokalemia
Isoproterenol Supplied: 1 mg/mL in 1-mL vials IV infusion: Mix 1 mg in 250 mL NS, LR, or D5W	Significant bradycardia (temporary therapy only) Torsades de pointes	Infusion: 2 ug/min to 10 ug/min	Can exacerbate ischemia and arrhythmias (PVCs, VT) Increases cardiac output and myocardial work Not indicated in cardiac arrest or hypotension **Do not mix with epinephrine!**
IV fluids	1. Expand blood volume 2. Keep IV lines patent	IV lines: Normal saline or lactated Ringer's preferred, but may use D5W	Do not give fluids without indication of volume depletion Monitor for overload
Lidocaine Supplied: Preloaded 20 mg/mL in 5-mL syringes; also: 10 mg/mL in 5-mL vials in 5-mL vials (total = 50 mg) Can be given via ET tube **Magnesium sulfate** Supplied: 10-mL ampules of 50% MgSO4 = 5 gm of magnesium; 2-mL ampules: (total = 1 gm/2 mL)	1. Ventricular ectopy (PVCs) 2. VF 3. VT 4. Wide-complex PSVT or tachyarrhythmias of uncertain type Magnesium deficiency, which is associated with cardiac arrhythmias	Bolus: 1.0 mg/kg to 1.5 mg/kg with additional bolus of 0.5 mg/kg to 1.5 mg/kg every 5 to 10 min as needed until 3 mg/kg total Infusion: 2 mg/min to 4 mg/min (mix 1 gm in 500 mL of D5W) Load: 1 g to 2 g mixed in 50 mL to 100 mL of D5W and given over 5 to 60 min Infusion: 0.5 g to 1.0 g (4 mEq to 8 mEq) per hour for up to 24 hours	Confusion Agitation Heart block Decrease dose after 24 hours or monitor levels Reduce second dose 50% in CHF, acute MI, liver failure, the elderly, and in patients with shock Do not use in bradycardiac-related PVCs Monitor blood levels Drowsiness Respiratory depression

ACLS Adult Drug Chart (continued)

Drug	Use	Dosage	Complications
Morphine Supplied: 2 to 5 mg/mL in 1-mL syringes	1. Acute MI pain 2. Pulmonary edema	1 mg to 3 mg IV every 5 min as needed	Decreased respiratory drive Nausea and vomiting Hypotension Avoid use in head-injury patients
Nitroglycerin Supplied: SL tablets: 0.3, 0.4 mg Inhaler: 0.4 mg/dose Ampules: 5 mg in 10 mL 8 mg in 10 mL 10 mg in 10 mL	1. Angina 2. CHF associated with acute MI 3. Hypertension (IV use)	0.3 or 0.4 mg sublingually and repeat Q 3 to 5 min for a total of 3 tabs Infusion: 10 µg/min to 20 µg/min and increase by 5 µg/min to 10 µg/min Q 5 to 10 min (mix 50 or 100 mg in 250 mL D5W or saline)	Hypotension Headache Flushing Tachycardia Pardoxical bradyccardia Avoid use in glaucoma, hypotension, and suspected tamponade
Norepinephrine Supplied: 1 mg/mL in 4-mL ampules Mix 4 mg in 250 mL D5W or D5NS. Avoid diluting in NS alone.	1. Severe hypotension 2. Shock	Infusion: 0.5 µg/min to 1.0 µg/min Refractory shock: 8 ug/min to 30 µg/min	Increased vasoconstriction Severe headaches Increased myocardial oxygen consumption Do not administer in same line as alkaline solutions Relatively contraindicated in hypovolemic patients Administer through central access
Oxygen	1. Ischemia 2. Hypoxemia 3. Cardiac arrest	Highest concentration possible; 100% via ET tube	Rare: oxygen toxicity Use concentration of 24% to 35% in patients with COPD

From *Easy ACLS: Advanced Cardiac Life Support Preparatory Manual* by Andrew D. Weinberg and James L. Paturas. Copyright © 1995 by Jones and Bartlett Publishers, Inc.

ACLS Adult Drug Chart (continued)

Drug	Use	Dosage	Complications
Procainamide Supplied: 100 mg/mL in 10-mL vials (total = 8 g) 500 mg/mL in 2-mL vials (total = 1 g)	1. Suppression of PVCS and recurrent VT when lidocaine contra-indicated or failed 2. Acceptable for wide-complex tachycardias indistinguishable from VT	Infusion: 20 mg/min until: 1. 17 mg/kg total given 2. QRS widens more than 50% 3. Hypotension develops 4. Arrhythmia suppressed Maintenance: 1 mg/min to 4 mg/min (mix 1 g in 250 mL D5W)	QRS widening Hypotension AV block CNS depression Reduce dose and monitor levels in renal failure Avoid in patients with prolonged QT, digitalis toxicity, and torsades de pointes
Sodium bicarbonate Supplied: 50-mL preloaded syringe (8.4% sodium bicarbonate at 50 mEq/50 mL)	1. Metabolic acidosis 2. Beneficial in patients with pre-existing hyperkalemia	1 mEq/kg as initial dose, then half every 10 min Use ABGs to guide all therapy	Alkalosis Electrolyte abnormalities (e.g.,hypokalemia) Avoid use in hypokalemic patients
Sodium nitroprusside Supplied: 10 mg/mL in 5-mL vials (total = 50 mg)	1. Hypertension 2. Heart failure	Infusion: 0.1 to 5 μg/kg/min (mix 50 mg to 100 mg in 250 mL D5W) Light sensitive: Cover IV bag with opaque material	Hypotension, reflex tachycardia, angina Decrease dose in renal or liver failure Monitor for cyanide toxicity (blood levels)
Verapamil and Diltiazem Supplied: *Verapamil:* 2.5 mg/mL in 2-4-, and 5-mL vials (totals = 5, 10, and 12.5 mg) *Diltiazem:* 5 mg/mL in 5- or 10-mL vials (totals = 25 or 50 mg)	Control ventricular response in 1. Atrial flutter 2. Atrial fibrillation 3. Multifocal atrial tachycardia 4. Other SVTs 5. Narrow-complex PSVTs (Note: adenosine is drug of choice)	*Verapamil:* 2.5 mg to 5 mg IV over 2 min Repeat doses of 5 mg to 10 mg every 15 to 30 min to a maximum of 20 mg *Diltiazem:* 0.25 mg/kg followed by a second dose of 0.35 mg/kg In atrial fibrillation, infusion of 5 to 15 mg/hr may be used	Decrease myocardial contractility in patients with LV dysfunction Exacerbate CHF in patients with LV dysfunction Hypotension AV block Nausea/vomiting

From *Easy ACLS: Advanced Cardiac Life Support Preparatory Manual* by Andrew D. Weinberg and James L. Paturas. Copyright © 1995 by Jones and Bartlett Publishers, Inc.